NEW SCIENCE LIBRARY

presents traditional topics from a modern perspective, particularly those associated with the hard sciences—physics, biology, and medicine—and those of the human sciences—psychology, sociology, and philosophy.

The aim of this series is the enrichment of both the scientific and spiritual view of the world through their mutual dialogue and exchange.

New Science Library is an imprint of Shambhala Publications.

General editor/Ken Wilber

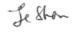

Imagery
in Healing: Shamanism
and Modern Medicine

Jeanne Achterberg

NEW SCIENCE LIBRARY
Shambhala
Boston and London
1985

NEW SCIENCE LIBRARY
An imprint of Shambhala Publications, Inc.
314 Dartmouth Street
Boston, Massachusetts 02116

*Distributed in the United States by Random House
and in Canada by Random House of Canada Ltd.*
Printed in the United States of America

Library of Congress Cataloging in Publication Data

Achterberg, Jeanne, 1942—
  Imagery in healing
  Bibliography: p.
  Includes index.
  1. Medicine and psychology.   2. Mind and body.
3. Imagery (Psychology)   4. Medicine, Psychosomatic.
I. Title.
R726.5.A24   1985   615.5   84–20748
ISBN 0–87773–307–4
ISBN 0–394–73031–3 (Random House)

Design / Eje Wray
Typesetting / G&S Typesetters / Austin, Texas in Linotron Palatino

Contents

Acknowledgments

This book belongs to Frank Lawlis, my husband, who sired it in every sense. It was a matter of circumstance that I became the scribe for the adventure. The journeys through the shaman's world, the teasing out of scientific principles to support the data we'd gathered, the clinical replications of material that ranged far afield from contemporary psychology and medicine—all are part of our close personal and professional relationship. He is first and foremost a scientist, as am I. The shaman's role was mutually donned in pursuit of the depths of scientific discovery. And, in as much as I respect his fine skills as a statistician and his sensitive judgments as a clinician, I am likewise able to feel confident in my own similar observations. We give each other courage and support to move out into the unsanctioned regions of consciousness, and confidence that the direction is good.

I would very much like to thank those people who made space in their lives over the past several years, so that I could have the luxury of researching and writing. I will always have fond memories of writing fervently to meet the deadlines, looking up periodically to see the seasons change in our beautiful woods. The time has truly been a gift.

My children should be thanked for their special contributions: Barry, who kept me in tune with the present and tolerated my absent-mindedness in the tasks of daily living, and Lee Ann, who took on the tedious, unrewarding task of working on the book's bibliography. Also, the manuscript review work and general emotional support of Barbara Peavey and Maggie Marrero were greatly appreciated.

My gratitude is expressed to the faculty and resources of the Department of Rehabilitation Science. In many ways, the department remains a stronghold of classic—but, unfortunately, rare—academic freedom. In dealing with people who are often regarded as hopeless cases, with people whose lives are completely altered by their physical disability, no direction of thought that might improve the human condition is considered an improper inquiry. The students have been especially helpful in their willingness to listen, offer comments, and read sections of the manuscript. Nan Wells and David Casey are to be commended for their extended efforts.

Three people deserve mention as major influences, not only on my work, but I believe also on the direction of the cultural evolution. First, I learned from Huston Smith, philosopher and master teacher, how necessary it is to look beyond the petty differences of doctrine for the threads of truth and validity in the spiritual viewpoint, and, indeed, how we as scientists cannot escape the relevancy of that viewpoint in plying our trade. Second, in countless instances over the past decade, I've taken a jog in my personal path, or a new turn in my research, and looked backward in time only to see Larry LeShan already there, glasses hung about his neck, chuckling, swinging his machete mind to blaze the trail. And finally, Michael Harner entered our lives most recently and has helped pull many of the pieces together with his wonderful, experiential, academic approach to ancient ways. And from all of them, I've learned maybe the most important lesson of all: the need to be able to find humor in the Divine Order.

A very special acknowledgment is due to Virginia Hine, dear friend and mentor, whose gently felt presence continues its great influence on my thoughts. The concept for the book arose out of night-long discussions and scores of letters, which had nothing overtly to do with science or shamans or medicine, or so we thought. Rather, they had to do with relationships between people who sensed a special love for each other, as Frank and I did, and as she and her husband had. We called it a holobond, and a network of likeminded souls formed, with Virginia—ever the cultural anthropologist—at the helm. The painful, ecstatic unfolding and enfolding of oneself into the other person and back, the recognition of having been cut from the same fabric and knowing full well an eternal inseparability led all of us to reexamine our personal views of reality. Hints of the texture of this enormous perplexity came to us through myths and legends, the great spiritual teachings, and new developments in science. The material herein was found as a vital part of that exploration.

Imagery in Healing

Introduction

Imagery has always played a key role in medicine. What is imagery? Imagery is the thought process that invokes and uses the senses: vision, audition, smell, taste, the senses of movement, position, and touch. It is the communication mechanism between perception, emotion and bodily change. A major cause of both health and sickness, the image is the world's oldest and greatest healing resource.

Imagery, or the stuff of the imagination, affects the body intimately on both seemingly mundane and profound levels. Memories of a lover's scent call forth the biochemistry of emotion. The mental rehearsal of a sales presentation or a marathon race evokes muscular change and more: blood pressure goes up, brain waves change, and sweat glands become active. Because of this pronounced effect the image has on the body, it yields power over life and death, and plays a key role in the less dramatic aspects of living as well.

In primitive societies, the witch doctor shakes the bones and utters a curse. The victim's heart flutters, his temperature drops, and death comes quickly. An autopsy would show that the hex had the effect of causing the body to shut down—a parasympathetic nervous system death, the physiologists might call it. The victim dies, not from fright, but from hopelessness, from the vivid working of the imagination.

A terminally ill cancer patient goes to the shrine at Lourdes, France. A woman with severe rheumatoid arthritis crosses the border into Mexico to get therapy that is unproven according to U.S. authorities and therefore illegal in this country. A couple, long childless, pays a first visit to a famous medical school's infertility clinic. In each of the cases, positive changes in the condition in question have been documented that either preceded treatment or accompanied what might be classified as medically worthless intervention. Patients all over the world are administered placebos of one kind or another. Often they show decreases in pain, nausea, anxiety, and even in tumor cells. It is not just their attitude that changes; their biochemistry has also undergone a transformation. Far from being the duping of innocents and malingerers, placebos and the power of suggestion tend to work best in people who need and want to get well.

The common feature of these events—the mental rehearsals, the voodoo curses, visits to religious or medical shrines and response to placebos—is that they all serve to alter the *images* or the expectancy that the persons hold regarding the state of their health. And in doing so, the images cause profound physiological change, a fact that must not be obscured by the glamor of modern medicine. Regardless of technological advancement, we will always have to contend with this vast complex of expectancies, beliefs, motivations, and the sometimes belligerent, sometimes miraculous, role of the imagination.

There is little argument about the negative power of the imagination on health. Acceptance for the idea no doubt stems from widely publicized research on stress and disease, as well as personal observation and intuition. Most people seem to have acknowledged at least a tentative connection between causal factors emanating from their state of mind and the subsequent observation of colds or infection or other evidence of diminished resistance to disease. What has not been proposed often in modern times is that the reverse must also be true. Since nature creates few one-way passages, if we can become ill through our misbehaviors, even die from hexes and broken hearts, then we must also be able to make ourselves well.

A renewal of focus on the imagination as at once an ancient and potent aspect of healing will help mark this decade as having initiated the most dramatic advances in medicine the world has yet seen. The forces responsible for bringing about these changes represent a grand confluence of theology, psychology, medicine, and anthropology, and are embodied in the personages of the scientist and the shaman.

This celebration of consciousness, of the power of the human psyche, and of the imagination as the essence of the universe, is gaining momentum even in unlikely academic circles. Medicine is not the target, nor even the cause of these great changes; but it is a beneficiary nonetheless. Nowhere is there such a concrete manifestation of the illusionary stuff that is mind and soul as in the human body. It is there, in the body, in its state of relative health or sickness, that the harmony of the person with the cosmos is portrayed. The body has no secrets; it never lies. Neither the sins of omission and commission in the environment, nor past and present thoughts, can pass without leaving their corporeal mark. The treatment of this complex landscape of thinking, feeling and being has been the province of medicine, for better or for worse. And so it is on the field of medicine that the new developments, the new understandings of the powers of the imagination, will have their most directed force.

Definite themes have emerged from the study of the imagination as healer, which relate to two basic ways the image is believed to positively impact upon health. First is what I have called *preverbal* imagery. Here, the imagination acts upon one's own physical being. Images communicate with tissues and organs, even cells, to effect a change. The communication can be deliberate or not. It is preverbal in the sense that it probably evolved much earlier than language, and uses different neural pathways for the transmission of information. The second type of healing imagery is *transpersonal*, embodying the assumption that information can be transmitted from the consciousness of one person to the physical substrate of others.

The scientific method is currently far more applicable to the study of the preverbal type of imagery. The preverbal phenomena can be described using facts derived from physiology, anatomy, chemistry, and the behavioral sciences. The proposition can, and has been, tested using the scientific method. Transpersonal imagery, on the other hand, requires the existence of channels of information flow that have not been identified by the tools of science. The validation of transpersonal imagery must therefore be sought in the more qualitative types of observational data gathered by the anthropologists, theologians, medical historians, and others, as well as by intuitive, philosophical speculation. The greatest support for this theory comes from the tenacity with which humans have clung to a belief in transpersonal healing, and have been reinforced in that belief system, for at least 20,000 years.

Although the dichotomy of imagery into transpersonal and preverbal modes is useful in describing and understanding healing systems, it is only grossly correct. The two types intermingle conceptually and in practice, and there is a considerable amount of variance in the application of both. The complexity of describing the image does not end in its categorization, however. In the following pages appears an unlikely mixture of art and science, history and medicine. As might be expected in the search for knowledge of one of the great enigmas of human nature, uncovering the dimensions of the imagination has required traveling along multiple avenues. Some were frankly bizarre, others offered only tenuous leads, still others were so enchanting it was difficult to move away at all. This book is the story of my search—spiraling around the idea of the imagination as healer, weaving in threads of metaphor, touching time and again on the primacy of consciousness as a fact of human existence.

I will begin in Chapter 1 by telling the story of the shamans— trying to treat their perspective appropriately, but with a scientific eye. In describing the imagination and healing, it seemed logi- cal to approach the knowledge of these long-recognized experts. Shamanism *is* the medicine of the imagination. The shaman is ubiq- uitous throughout time, throughout the world. Shamanism is and has been the most widely practiced type of medicine on the planet, particularly for serious illness. The shamans are the ones who are said to understand, in a spiritual sense, the nexus of the mind, the body, and the soul. Their chief task has always been to heal their people of the ills of humanity—whatever form those maladies might assume. The shamans claim to have special skills for journeying to the planes of the imagination where healing the body and healing the planet are possible.

Most of the shamanic lore is so foreign to the myths of contem- porary medicine that it has long been discarded as too fanciful, too untenable for twentieth-century, sensible, civilized, rational human- kind. Nevertheless, shamanic health practices have continued to thrive (or at least survive) alongside of the mainstream of medical thought.

The traditional concept of shamanism would place it within the classification of transpersonal healing, and it is upon that issue that the shamans have established their reputation. However, preverbal imagery plays a strong role, as well. The shamans' ritual work has a direct therapeutic effect on the patient by creating vivid images, and by inducing altered states of consciousness conducive to self- healing. Too, the shamanic concepts of disease and the community involvement in healing deserve consideration in these times when disease has become an entity apart from its host and from the en- vironmental circumstances.

In Chapter 2, the qualitative, historical evidence for the imagina- tion as a healing tool is explored further, specifically as it is found firmly embedded in the lineage of Western medicine. Asclepius, Aristotle, Galen, and Hippocrates, regarded as the fathers of medicine, used imagery for both diagnosis and therapy. Their sensitive observations concerning the ability of the image to cure as well as kill provided a legacy that was fully realized by the creative physicians of the Renaissance.

Because we are all significantly influenced by the Anglo-Saxon heritage, I have included a discussion of those healing traditions of England and Europe that reflected upon the imagination. For several hundred years, the Catholic church functioned as the authority in matters of health. The treatments the Church sanctioned were pilgrimages and rituals that still bore the pagan taint of shamanism, although the gods differed. The early and medieval Church incorporated the ancient Greek methods of healing in special temples dedicated to the premise that vision and dreams contained seeds of knowledge regarding health.

Several scholars feel the true roots of shamanism in Western civilization lie in the practices of the wise women, who were considered the ultimate purveyors of the supernatural, and hence, of the imagination. In Celtic times they were priestesses, but their successors were condemned as witches. The ebb and ultimate dissolution of women's influence on medicine and science were pivotal in directing healing away from the classic womanly virtues of nurturance, intuition, empathy, and emotionality—all seen as threats and impediments to progress of the new scientific order. Their specific knowledges, however, were borrowed and sustained for generations by physicians, quacks, and the Church alike.

This history of health practices is fascinating in and of itself, but more important, it provides us with ground; it tells us that the imagination has always been an integral part of the healing process, regardless of cultural disguise. In each instance of history, the gifts of the imagination took primacy over pharmacy and surgery, and those who were skilled at wielding the powers of the image were awarded the greatest stature in the healing hierarchy. The scientific age brought this acclaim to a screeching halt.

It has only recently become quasi-respectable again to ask (and answer) questions about the mind and medicine. Chapter 3 describes the work of those who are involved in such query, and who might best be called shaman/scientists. They were and are in the midst of mainline medicine, and have combined the ancient wisdoms with modern technology. For the most part, these practitioners are no strangers to the terrain of the spirit, and with their help, the humanistic, naturalistic practices are gradually returning from the fringes of medicine.

From subject matter as diverse as hypnosis, autogenics, biofeedback, general medical practice, and the placebo response, it is apparent that the imagination enters health care in ways not dissimilar to those described in the history of healing. First, it is a part of all health care, in the sense that every interaction with health care personnel, every diagnosis and treatment, creates some kind of an image in the patient's mind. These images, in and of themselves, can turn the course of the disease. Second, imagery is once again being used as diagnosis. Because of their intimate contact with the physical body, images appear to express a body wisdom, an understanding of both the status and prognosis of health. Third, imagery is used as therapy—its most controversial application. And finally, the imagination is employed to systematically rehearse anxiety-provoking events such as natural childbirth and the painful treatment for severe burns.

Before moving on to the innovative research and practice that will likely become the foundation for the medicine of the future, I relate evidence for the imagination and health, told from the special vantage place of the scientist. The scientific findings by no means explain away the effectiveness of the imagination in health, but rather describe the events in different ways. The study of the imagination, involving as it does the external verification of intrinsic, private events, is especially susceptible to the whimsical nature of personal need, as well as the foibles of human beings in reporting such events. Therefore, the scientific method is not only necessary, but absolutely critical for establishing accurate, replicable, valid information, which can be used in a productive sense in health. Science, when well practiced, is a ballet of discovery, an elegant accoutrement to the rest of the world's knowledge. More important, it provides a prohibition on self-delusion, which distinguishes the scientific methods of observation from other ways of seeking information.

Even with the safeguards of the scientific methods, the descriptions the scientist (as well as the shaman) gives of the imagination and the healing process are myths. Scientists, artists, mystics, and poets still use their own special media to describe the imagination. They paint pictures on the canvas of their choice. The stories that come from science are no more nor less true than those from the great traditions of culture, but they are different in both the methods used to obtain and view the data, and the level at which the description is given. Using information from the basic sciences, in

Chapter 4 I have provided a description of the transition of mental images into physical change—or mind into matter, as some would have it. While the answers are clearly not all in, enough information is available from neuroanatomy and physiology, as well as biochemistry, to substantiate the existence of the pathways. Images, indeed all thoughts, are electrochemical events, which are intricately woven into the fabric of the brain and the body.

In considering science and the imagination, we are confronted with the facts of differing levels of description, all obtained with the scientific method. The behavioral and social sciences, too, have studied the function of the imagination in healing systems, but in terms of the behavior of the individual, and within the context of the social milieu. Their position deserves note, and is outlined in Chapter 5. Rather than considering the imagination in either a mystical sense (as the shamans would) or as a physiological, biochemical phenomena, it becomes a hypothetical construct, a nonthing, which is measured only through the observable behavior of persons and their societies. Analysis of the image tends to revolve around psychological, rather than physiological, events. Because of these scientists, we realize the important distinction between illness and disease, with the former being the unique personal impact of mental or physical pathology, and the latter being the pathology itself. Techniques that use the imagination to achieve health are most likely regarded as affecting the illness, but not necessarily the disease. From the behavioral scientists, particularly, comes a wealth of experimental work and studied application of the imagination as therapy in psychological disorders.

In Chapter 6, I have concluded with information on the frontier of health: the field of immunology. As more and more is known of this magnificent system of defense, it appears the major diseases of humanity could be conquered if the immune system could be trained to function effectively. Diseases of the immune system include cancer, allergies, infections, the autoimmune disorders such as multiple sclerosis and rheumatoid arthritis, and a multitude of other conditions that are a consequence of either a sluggish or a hyperactive immune system.

We have a thirty-year research effort from scientists such as Walter Cannon, Hans Selye, and many others, showing the potential for stress to hamper the immune function. There are series after series of animal trials from the most respected laboratories in the world showing that under stressed conditions, the compromised immune system can result in disease or even death. We even have growing acceptance for the notion that stress exacerbates the growth of cancer in humans, triggers flare-ups in patients with rheumatoid arthritis, and sends asthmatics off to the emergency room for oxygen. Stress is implicated as a factor in both onset and exacerbation of all of the autoimmune diseases—those conditions where the immune system can no longer discriminate self from nonself, friend from foe.

Fortunately, even though the immune system is violently assaulted by many types of behaviors and thoughts, there is information that it can also be enhanced and programmed through conscious acts. According to new research, a variety of techniques—specific images, positive feelings, suggestions, learning to respond to stressors in a relaxed way—all have the potential for increasing the ability of the immune system to counter disease. Very current studies have shown that the immune system itself is under the direct control of the central nervous system, particularly those areas of the brain implicated in the transmission of the image to the body.

A profound relationship exists between the brain, behavior, psychological factors, and the immune system, although the exact nature of the relationship has yet to be specified. New behavioral therapies that highlight the imagination, such as guided imagery, hypnosis, biofeedback—all with a distinct tinge of shamanism—have been shown to influence immunology under controlled testing situations.

There is drama, here, as the elusive mysteries of the human mind begin to unfold—drama unparalleled on the battlefield, or in space, or in politics, or in any other arena. The scientific paradigm shifts, the metaphors blend. It is a good time to be alive.

The Shaman: Master Healer of the Imaginary Realms

I don't know what you learned from books, but the most important thing I learned from my grandfathers was that there is a part of the mind that we don't really know about and that it is that part that is most important in whether we become sick or remain well.

Thomas Largewhiskers, 100-year-old Navaho medicine man

The shamans' work is conducted in the realm of the imagination, and their expertise in using that terrain for the benefit of the community has been recognized throughout recorded history. "The limitations of time and space are transcended. . . . Rocks and stones speak. Men turn into animals and animals into men. It is a world replete with archaic symbolism, in which the shaman journeys the breadth of the universe or around the moon on missions of utmost importance to his people."[1] Since the dawn of civilization, these voyages have been conducted to experience the Creator, to seek wisdom, and to heal the ailments of the body. I will focus upon the healing aspect here, describing the phenomenon in the allegory of the shaman and of the scientist.

If healing with the imagination is ever to have an impact on the practice of modern medicine, it must first be measured and described with the yardsticks of science. On the other hand, we must not ignore the shamans' own wisdom. The shamans tend to believe that Western explanations of their medicine are either grossly offensive, or bordering on just plain foolish. According to Bergman in his description of the Navaho, the shamans' explanations of why their medicine works, "should they feel like giving any, tend to be unsatisfying to us since they are based on the supernatural."[2] Shamanistic medicine should not be robbed of its significance by pretending that it is something that it is not, or by regarding it as a bastardized, primitive form of medical and psychological aid designed to pacify the ignorant natives. It is probably not too harmful to call what the shamans do "psychotherapy," or an outlet for aberrant personalities, or to say, at best, they provide a basis for the networking of the community. This labeling might promote good will toward the preservation of these ancient practices. However, the paths of the shaman are first and foremost spiritual. It is here, as "technicians of the sacred"[3] that their expertise resides, and here where their success is measured by their own cultures' yardsticks.

The current widespread interest in the shamanic practices, often manifested as an uncritical reverence for anything loosely affiliated with native culture, surely must reflect a longing for a more humanistic, spiritual inclusion in modern medicine. One might say that the Medicine Wheel of Western civilization has looked to the North far too long now, having much knowledge but little feeling.

What is Shamanism?

Shaman is a word derived from the Russian *saman*. Weston La Barre, a distinguished professor of anthropology at Duke University, notes that the shaman is the world's oldest professional, and the personage from whom both the modern doctor and priest descend. "The shaman was the original artist, dancer, musician, singer, dramatist, intellectual, poet, bard, ambassador, advisor of chiefs and kings, entertainer, actor and clown, curer, stage magician, juggler, jongleur, folksinger, weatherman, artisan, culture hero and trickster-transformer."[4] Mircea Eliade, an author of classic anthropological and theological works, has reviewed the vast literature on shamanism, and finds the shamans characterized as priest, physician, magician, sorcerer, exorcist, political leader, psychotic and mountebank.[5]

The popular concept of shamanism typically relates to the practice of any sort of nonmedical, folk, or mentalistic healing, or to any health system that does not incorporate Western medicine. The words *witch doctor* and *medicine man* are often used interchangeably, with *shaman*, but this is an incorrect understanding. A shaman may well have an herbal lore or a knowledge of crisis or trauma medicine, but, in the stricter anthropological sense, shamans are those individuals who distinguish themselves through particular practices of ecstasy or altered states of consciousness. During these states, they ascend to the sky or descend to the underworld of the imagination. The focus of the shamanic journeying is on obtaining power or knowledge in order to help the community, or on healing—although disease, and hence, cure, may be quite unlike what might be recognized as such in conventional medicine.

Eliade and others view shamanism as a healing system involving techniques for entering into and interpreting the landscape of the imagination that is encountered during the journeying, or the "magical flight."[6] The achievement of a state of ecstasy (or trance, or altered state of consciousness) is agreed upon as a universal aspect of shamanic practice, but certainly not every ecstatic would be considered a shaman. Indeed, the shamanic ecstasy has been identified as a highly specific, special category of altered state, one that can be entered into and exited from at will.[7]

In addition, the shaman is identified as one who has guardian spirits (also sometimes called power animals, helping spirits, tutelaries, totems, or fetishes), from whom power and knowledge is gained. Not everyone who claims these spirits is a shaman, however, and laypersons may have similar spirits who have not conferred shamanic power upon them, or they may be in possession of lesser spirits, or just fewer of them.[8] While the spirits offer protection to the layperson and shaman alike, the use of them to heal others or for divination is normally the province of the shaman alone.[9]

The shaman, then, is defined both by practices and intent: Shamanic practice involves the ability to move in and out of a special state of consciousness, a notion of a guardian spirit complex, and has the purpose of helping others.[10] The most distinguishing feature of shamanic work for the purposes of the current treatise is that the shamans have been recognized throughout the recorded history of the human species as having the ability to heal with the imagination, par excellence.

The Shaman in the Traditional Healing Complex

The healing techniques of the shaman have always existed side-by-side with medicine of a more mechanical or technological nature. A good shaman, noting that the patient had an arrow sticking out between his shoulder blades, would not likely have ordered up an altered state of consciousness at least until the intrusion was removed, available medicines were applied to staunch the bleeding, and others used to halt infection and pain. The skill level for these tasks might be considerable, but nothing compared to what must come next: the determination of the power base of the patient and the enemy, an examination of motives and belief systems, and an interpretation of the trauma in the cultural context. All of this was the work of the shaman.

The shamans, performing the difficult tasks of seeking the connectedness of all things and protecting the souls of the sick and dying, have traditionally been used as treatment of the last resort. For simple problems, nature has provided the obvious remedies, widely sown across the planet and well-known to early cultures. The aches of being alive could be relieved by willow bark, the forerunner of today's aspirin; the pains of dying were alleviated by the essence of the poppy. Even menstrual cramps and irregularities could be reduced by plants that grow in every fertile niche of the earth. Infections could be halted, fevers lowered, and madness constrained by nature's offerings.

Mechanical maneuverings of the contents of the human frame were also not beyond the skill level of even the very early humans. Brain surgery has been successfully conducted for at least ten-thousand years: skulls from the period show careful removal and replacement of bony material, and indications that the patient lived to die from other causes.[11] Bones from the Paleolithic, Mesolithic, and Neolithic periods suggest that prehistoric humans were able to keep themselves alive for about forty years, and sundry well-healed wounds have been noted. Ears and noses have been replaced using delicate plastic surgery for at least two-thousand years.[12]

The removal of offending bodies (bullets, tumors, slivers and ingrown toenails) tends to require a good eye and a steady hand, but a philosophical nature is optional. Mechanical medicine, like plumbing and electronics, depends upon knowledge of the circuitry, but not necessarily an appreciation for how a toilet or a radio (or a human) fits into the cosmos. Typically in shamanic cultures, a healing hierarchy exists, with those whose singular talent rests in physical manipulation or prescription at the bottom, followed by specialists in diagnosis, and then crowned by the shamans and their use of the imagination to intervene with the supernatural.

There is a fourth category of persons in this hierarchy that also has the reputation of working with the imagination in powerful ways: their name is sometimes improperly translated into English as "witch." These folk delve into the dark side of magic, and are called upon when the shaman's medicine fails, particularly if the disease is believed to be the result of a hex. Needless to say, their power is greatly feared, and they are believed to be able, and certainly willing, to call up evil forces of destruction. The documented instances of "voodoo death" and hexing in American medical journals attests to their ability to create malevolent outcomes through the workings of the imagination.[13]

The shaman may have knowledge and function in several healing roles. It would be unthinkable, however, to go to a bone setter who was not also a shaman to ask how to live a life, or for an interpretation of the meaning of a disease in a cultural context. The distinction between mechanical, technological medicine and shamanic medicine seems to have been clear until recent times, with the former having always had a stellar role in relieving the torment of physical suffering. In these modern times, medicine as technology has been beset with high expectations. In the first instance, it is regarded as exclusive medicine, ignoring the significant, ancient and ongoing contribution of the shaman's wisdom toward total health. And in the second, ironically, the medical doctor, him/herself, has been cloaked in the myth of the shaman as omnipotent healer— an amazingly inaccurate perception considering the lack of training (and inclination) on the part of the physician for the ancient shamanic practice.

The Ancient Way

Shamanism is the oldest and most widespread method of healing with the imagination. There is archaeological evidence suggesting that the techniques of the shaman are at least 20,000 years old, with vivid evidence of their antiquity in the cave paintings in the south of France. In Les Trois Freres cave, there is a mysterious, partly carved, partly painted deerlike creature thought to represent a shaman. Carvings on reindeer bones from the Paleolithic period showing the shaman garbed in an animal mask were found in Pin Hole Cave in England. Another reindeer bone carving of enormous interest shows a pregnant woman lying underneath a deer, presumably to garner strength for her ordeal. (The highly prevalent deer motif as healing spirit will be discussed in other contexts in this chapter.) LeBarre summarizes the anthropological evidence for dating the shamanic complex to the Paleolithic *Ur-kultur*, and in his opinion, shamanism is the Ur-religion and the essence of all supernatural religions.[14] (The *Ur-kultur* spread with human groups to all parts of the earth, and is still visible in some cultural practices.)

The practices of shamans are remarkably similar in Asia, Australia, Africa, the Americas, and even in Europe. This consistency leads to widespread speculation about earlier contacts among the people of these lands. Harner, however, questions why these practices would be passed down for 20,000 some odd years, when other aspects of the various social systems are in great contrast. He suggests it is because shamanism works, and, through trial and error, the same techniques for healing were adopted by diverse populations. He also believes that one need not share the cultural perspective of the shaman in order for shamanism to be effective. "The ancient way is powerful, and taps so deeply into the human mind, that one's usual cultural belief systems and assumptions about reality are essentially irrelevant." [15] In other words, belief in the invariant laws of the universe called forth in shamanic practice is no more necessary to make them work than a belief in gravity is necessary to make objects fall to the ground. In this context of the shamanic tradition, we can conceive of a natural environ that responds when we call Her in the old ways She has learned to understand. We are dealing with a classically conditioned universe, if you will. This position of Harners' is consonant with the shamans' explanation of how their own system works, and explains why common elements can be observed in all parts of the world.

Sociologists and those of psychiatric persuasion, however, normally take another point of view toward shamanism or any nonmedical healing. This view maintains that any benefit derived from such healing systems is highly specific to the world view held by the culture, and that one would not, therefore, expect any cross-cultural healing to occur unless there were chance commonalities in ritual and symbol. Any similarities found from tribe to tribe would be explained by the mutual availability of raw materials to weave into ritual meaning; the physiology of human beings, which is intimately affected by their emotions; and the undeniable human need to harmonize inner conflict and be integrated with a group and a spirit world. Jerome Frank has been a well-respected spokesman for this line of reasoning, which leads to the conclusion that any effectiveness of shamanic healing is a function of heightened expectancy on the part of the sick and injured, and that the true benefit of the primitive techniques is to provide emotional relief and a sense of community. [16] This position would also assert that shamanism would be most successful for psychological problems (depression and anxiety), for diagnoses that fall within the traditional concept of "psychosomatic," and for conditions that stem from cultural or familial alienation, as opposed to "physical" disease as it is diagnosed by Western medical practitioners. We will discuss how these traditional distinctions between so-called psychosomatic and physical disease are currently breaking down in more detail in Chapter 5.

The Meaning of Health and Disease in the Shamanic System

It is important to consider the healing techniques of the imagination used by the shamans in the context of their usual belief structure concerning the nature of health and illness. In the discussion that follows, as well as in all generalizations about shamanistic practice, certain quirks of cultures will prove exceptions to the points being made. There are sufficient points of convergence across all traditions, however, to justify broad observations.

First and foremost, avoiding death is not the purpose for the practice of medicine in the shamanic traditions. Our Western mistrust of these systems often comes from the observation that shamanic healing may not have resulted in an extension of life. Healing, for the shaman, is a spiritual affair. Disease is considered to have origins in, and gains its meaning from, the spirit world. The purpose of life, itself, is to be indoctrinated and initiated into the visionary regions of the spirit, and to maintain oneself in concert with all things on earth and in the sky. To lose one's soul is the gravest occurrence of all, since it would eliminate any meaning from life, now and forever. Thus, the purpose of much shamanic healing is primarily to nurture and preserve the soul, and to protect it from eternal wandering.

Illness, as it is conceived of even in the modern sense, is regarded as something entering the body from without, something that needs to be removed or destroyed or protected against. In the shamanic system, however, the primary problem is not the external element, but the loss of personal power that permitted the intrusion in the first place, whether it be an arrow or an evil spirit. (The "poison dart" theory of the Nekematigi of Papua New Guinea is a case in point. Here some, though not all, disease is classified as sorcery and regarded as the result of the magical shooting of poisoned darts from the enemy.)[17] Therefore, shamanic treatment for all ailments first emphasizes augmenting the power of the sick person, and only secondly counteracting the power of the illness-producing agent. All medicines, including Western when available, are used for both stages. Actually, this is rather advanced thinking, since recent discoveries in medical science support a similar description of the disease process, a topic that will be treated in some depth in Chapter 6. To briefly summarize the issue, the so-called primary external causes of major illness—viruses, bacteria, and other invisible elements in the environment—are a threat to health only when a person's natural protective mantle develops a weakness.

In the tribal societies where shamanism has flourished, the practice of healing overlaps and is integrated with all of secular and sacred life—with prayer, farming, marriage, war, and taboo. Grossinger notes that the shaman cannot work exclusively in the context of disease; history provides no basis or technology for the isolation of disease from the rest of the human condition. The dangers of isolating one part of living from another are recognized, and there is little interest in merely lengthening life, but rather in restoring balance. He also observes, in defense of the holistic, shamanistic medicine, that when we treat disease as a concrete entity capable of technologic remediation, we lose the notion of an integrated system. The disease may manifest outwardly as pathological changes, "but it is also the place where all other crises and necessities of the organism come together. It is the most intimate writing of the turbulence and changes of life on the single bodies and collective body of the biosphere. Nothing else, except maybe dream or vision, forces the organism to reconcile itself instantaneously with the devastating pagan powers of which it is made." Illness, he says, tugs one toward the reality of both biological and social existence. Disease can lead to vision and personal growth, and in light of this, "the world of sterile chemicals and operating tables is a cruel reversal and a wasteful joke." [18]

In the shamanic traditions, as one might expect, there is a far greater emphasis on disturbances of the spirit than one finds in the medicine of industrialized countries. The shaman is well-skilled at differential diagnosis of spirit disorders. Sometimes the soul may be diagnosed as having been frightened, other times depressed, and worst of all, it may have exited itself altogether (known as *susto*, or "soul loss," among Spanish speaking cultures). Both physical and mental symptoms are characteristic of the different states, and are regarded as quite serious. Without intervention, the patient may well die without resolving the problem that caused the disease in the first place, and thus be doomed to an eternal life of being out of synchrony with the universe.

Any current thrust toward romanticizing shamanic medicine or folk medicine in general should be tempered with the knowledge that often the remedies prescribed were clearly wrong and harmful from the standpoint of physical well-being. Jilek-Aall describes birthing procedures dictated by custom in parts of Africa that defy the course of nature. The result is high infant mortality, and a high incidence of epilepsy—a disorder known to be related to birth trauma.[19] Other conditions of early tribal life, such as major debilitative illnesses from impure food and water resources, rampant parasitic infestation, and a limited life expectancy, were regarded as normal conditions of living. Our advanced technology in sanitary conditions and nutrition has significantly reduced those problems in industrialized countries. Even in cultures that still have shamanic activities, the imported health facilities seem to be regarded as the first-line stance against injury, infection, and endemic disease.[20]

Unfortunately, "civilization" has created new health problems in the stead of those that it has ameliorated. For example, in contemporary Western medicine, life's natural passages are viewed as deficiency diseases that require medical attention. Newborn babies, about-to-be mothers, menopausal women, and people who are simply experiencing old age are hospitalized and medicated as if pathology were present. Even marriage and death require the legal stamp of medical approval. Growth rituals in our society have been turned over to the health care system; thus, the natural maturation and fruition of human condition are regarded as sicknesses, and in need of intervention.

The shamans are pivotal figures in the rites of passage for their respective cultures in quite another way. Their wisdom is consulted in events that are believed critical to living, such as naming the infants, the vision quest or puberty rites that signify the beginnings of adult responsibility, and the ceremonial occasions of birth and marriage. This stands to reason in a shamanic culture, where the shaman, as well as being a healer, serves as a philosopher/priest who is privy to the supernatural.

The function of any society's health system is ultimately tied to the philosophical convictions that the members hold regarding the purpose of life itself. For the shamanic cultures, that purpose is spiritual development. Health is being in harmony with the world view. Health is an intuitive perception of the universe and all its inhabitants as being of one fabric. Health is maintaining communication with the animals and plants and minerals and stars. It is knowing death and life and seeing no difference. It is blending and melding, seeking solitude and seeking companionship to understand one's many selves. Unlike the more "modern" notions, in shamanic society health is not the absence of feeling; no more so is it the absence of pain. Health is seeking out all of the experiences of Creation and turning them over and over, feeling their texture and multiple meanings. Health is expanding beyond one's singular state of consciousness to experience the ripples and waves of the universe.

Who Becomes a Shaman?

Both men and women apparently have equal potential for shamanic practice, but in cultures where the demands of daily living are great and continuous on women, men may simply have more leisure time to engage in the lengthy shamanic training. The personal knowledge and power of the shaman are gained through many, many journeys into other realms of consciousness, and "years of shamanic experience are usually necessary to arrive at a high degree of knowledge of the cosmic puzzle."[21] So, motivation, willingness, and time to engage in a lengthy learning period are all prerequisites to enter this, the oldest of professions.

The practice of shamanism is always regarded as being fraught with grave risk to the life and well-being of the practitioner, and in some cases, women may be more able or willing to tread upon the supernatural territory. In China, one particularly dangerous aspect of shamanism, "soul raising," is almost always practiced by women. Kendall, in viewing recent work on Asian shamanism, notes that women on the outskirts of the Chinese family were the only ones that dared mediate with the ancestors, since they had very little to lose by engaging in such a fearsome task. When economic circumstances threw them back on their own resources, they used intuitive abilities in a supernatural application to "dodge the vicissitudes of a male-dominant society."[22] This was true in Europe, too, where economic opportunity for women who were not highly born ranged from scant to nonexistent until this century.

A long-standing debate has existed in anthropological writings on whether shamanism is a shelter for deranged personalities. This topic will be covered later, in the discussion of shamanism and schizophrenia. Also, since shamanic practice is highly developed in the circumpolar area, there has been some speculation that the shamanic trance and other behaviors may represent Arctic hysteria, and be a function of extreme cold, desert solitude, and sundry vitamin deficiencies. This explanation can be readily dismissed since similar shamanic practices occur in the tropics.[23] Others have suggested shamans exist because the society at large encourages oppressed categories of persons—usually women in Asian shamanism—to use divine inspiration as "an oblique redressive strategy."[24]

The basic skills requisite for the shaman include the ability to create an atmosphere of awe, of spiritual power and omniscience, and the endurance to sustain a performance that requires concentration for hours or even weeks.[25] Facility for shamanism is demonstrated through reporting on supernatural occurrences during the vision quest, having dreams full of message and precognition, or showing talents such as clairvoyance. The prospective candidate's behaviors tend to indicate a greater than usual facility for using the imagination, and/or a miraculous ability to recover from significant illness—hence, the notions of the "divine illness" and the "wounded healer" that are prevalent throughout the literature on shamanism.[26]

Disease and the Initiatory Call

Disease plays at least two roles in the shamanic choice of vocation. First, being afflicted with certain diseases may automatically include one in the ranks of potential shamans. In Siberia, for instance, having epilepsy or other nervous disorders is a clear indication of shamanic talent. Second, the initiatory call in which the vocation is revealed may come during an acute physical or mental crisis. This issue is discussed by Joan Halifax, who writes that the initiation often comes from a crisis of powerful illness involving an encounter with forces of decay and destruction. "Illness thus becomes the vehicle to a higher plane of consciousness."[27] She tells of Matsuwa, a Huichol shaman, who did not receive shamanhood until he lost his right hand and maimed his foot. Only upon the impending crisis did he recognize his powers.

An account of the initiation of an Avam-Samoyed shaman has it that a man, stricken with smallpox, remained unconscious for three days. On the third day he appeared so lifeless that he was nearly buried. He had visions of going down to hell where he was carried to an island upon which stood the Tree of the Lord of the Earth. The Lord gave him a branch of the tree with which to make a drum. Moving on in his imagination, he came to a mountain. Entering a cave, he saw a naked man who caught him, cut off his head, chopped up his body, and boiled the bits in a kettle for three years. After this time, his body was reassembled and covered with flesh. During his adventures, he met the evil shamans and the lords of epidemics who gave him instruction on the nature of disease. He was strengthened in the land of shamanesses, taught how to "read inside his head," to see mystically without his normal eyes, and how to understand the language of plants. When he awoke finally, or rather was resurrected, he could begin to shamanize.[28]

Even in the evaluation of contemporary medicine and science, the shamans chosen by way of physical disease had special powers. A person who survived smallpox, the most dreaded of all plagues, could live to walk among the ill and treat them with no fear of infection. Any brush with death from which a person emerged with knowledge of the encounter, as well as specialized immunity, should be a clear calling to healing. It is a fair assumption that the shamans were in possession of a magnificent set of white blood cells.

Death/Rebirth as a Recurrent Theme

Tales of frightening initiations are not unusual. These ordeals occur particularly during the ritual vision quests, when a vocation is sought after days of fasting and isolation. Thus the mettle and motivation of the would-be shamans are put to test. The underlying theme, again and again, is one of death and rebirth, with visions of physical dismemberment and reconstruction being quite common.

Jilek reports a contemporary instance of the death and rebirth myth played out in the ritual of initiation among the Salish Indians. These Indians believe the shamanic healing power is available to all and is a "divine compensation for the technological assets of white civilization." Those who are chosen to exercise the power are called spirit dancers, and are initiated over a several day period. During this time, according to one report, "You call a new dancer a baby because he is starting out his life again . . . he is helpless." According to another, "They [initiators] kill you as an evil person, they revive you to a new human being, that's why they club you, you just go and pass out, but you come back. . . ."[29]

The Salish shamanic initiation includes first a period of torture and deprivation: being clubbed, bitten, thrown about, immobilized, blindfolded, teased, starved. When the initiate "gets his song straight," or the slate that is the mind is wiped clean, the guardian spirit or power animal appears. This second phase of initiation is accompanied by significant physical activity: running barefoot in the snow, swimming in icy waters, dancing and drumming to exhaustion. During the indoctrination period, the Indians describe entering into blissful or trance states, which some have compared with alcohol intoxication and heroin use. Others state, "I was jumping three feet high and I had such a thrill, a terrific feeling as if you were floating, as if you were in the air. . . ." "It seems to me this power is like electricity; that's why I would not let anybody dance behind me. . . . It's a force that makes you dance, something like a shock . . . you just hear your song and the drums. . . ."[30]

The ceremonials of the Salish Indians are again being practiced, and the number of spirit dancers is growing each year. They were suppressed for nearly a century for fear they would threaten white man's religion and government. Now, the spirit dancing serves to reintegrate the alienated from their communities, and as a treatment for behavioral or psychophysiologic disorders. Jilek's data on the effectiveness of the dancing as a cure for alcoholism are impressive.

The Shamanic State of Consciousness

The shamanic state of consciousness (Harner's SSC) is the very essence of shamanism; and it is critical to the premise that the shaman is the past and present master of the imagination as healer. The shamans claim to be able to enter at will an unusual state of consciousness, one conducive to special problem-solving abilities. The shamanic rituals—the drums and monotonous chants, the fasting and sleeplessness—allow the shaman to slip into a dream-like state, somewhere between sleep and wakefulness, where vivid imagery experiences are possible.

Risse claims that in the state of consciousness used in shamanic healing, mental resources are employed that modern persons either no longer have access to or are not interested in using, in view of the current reliance upon coherent and rational conscious thought. For difficult problems, instead of turning to rationality, the shaman turns to inner experiences for solutions, using sensory memories, as well as abstractions and symbolisms. "He reviews his subconscious flow of pictures without the use of the critical powers activated by consciousness as well as the grid of causality, time, and space."[31] The shaman, in effect, is plugging into a data bank that can't be known in the normal, waking state of consciousness. A description of the SSC that allows external verification, reproducibility, and is reliable across observers, will be the closest that this generation of scientific technology will come to understanding how the workings of the shaman's imagination could possibly act upon another person for diagnosis and cure as claimed.

Carlos Castaneda, in the many stories of his initiation by Don Juan, the Yaqui shaman, makes a critical distinction between types of consciousness. That is, there is an ordinary reality (the ordinary state of consciousness, or OSC, as Harner calls it), and a nonordinary reality (the SSC).[32] The shamanistic healing journey is accomplished in the nonordinary reality. Negligence in making this distinction and in understanding all that the definitions imply has led to erroneous conclusions about shamanistic healing. The belief that shamans dealt primarily with psychiatric cases (thus using the imagination to heal only imaginary ailments), or that the shamans' skills were based upon trickery and hallucinations (i.e., the shamans were psychopathological themselves) is a failure on the part of the observer to understand the ramifications of differing states of consciousness.

For the shaman, there are varying levels of reality, and he/she exists in some form on all of them, often perceiving simultaneous existence on one or several planes. The shaman may be journeying in the SSC, but at the same time appearing alert, aware, and even lucid in the OSC.[33] The worlds of dreams or of fantasy are no less "real" than the one world that is perceived in the ordinary waking state of consciousness—only different. The shamans' treasure trove of information is approached and applied in a special state, or "place," that permits interactions among the living and not living, the animals, and literally all the particles of the universe. Amazing cross-cultural agreement exists for this point, enough to shame our Western souls for not earlier attempting to glean information from this medical school of the millennia.

People who are accustomed to thinking in terms of more than one reality, such as metaphysicists, some quantum physicists, and mystics, have no problem in understanding the implications of the shamanic consciousness. When thoughts are conceived of as things, or things as thoughts (or, more precisely, the inevitable, eternal interchange between mass and energy), then the shamanic system, as embodied in the special state of being, can be viewed as something beyond an exclusive conglomerate of superstitious behavior, dishonest quacks, and gullible, desperate patients. (It should go without saying, though, that crass fraud exists in all healing systems, including shamanism.)

The implications of the existence of a real, but nonordinary, reality should first be examined in terms of the rituals and symbols used in healing ceremonies. "Ritual" and "symbol" are concepts contemporary Western cultures hold dear as metaphorical, or as pretend acts and items. In the SSC, however, these become—they actually *are*—what the shaman says they represent. When a shaman dons the skin of his power animal and dances around the campfire, it is the power animal dancing in the SSC, not the man and a skin in some theatrical rendition. When the shaman sucks a bloody object out of an ailing patient's chest, or presses into the patient's gut and retrieves a spider and claims to have extracted the disease, the Western scientist tends to evaluate the magicianlike performance in ordinary reality's terms. Did the cure make the patient physically well? Was the "thing" gotten from the patient medically related to the disease?

Such questions are irrelevant to the shamanic sense of health. Getting well may have little or nothing to do with the body; and since there is not such a thing as a symbol, only the thing itself, the chicken gizzard or the blood-stained down are exactly what the shaman says they are—and that is whatever was revealed during the SSC. The symbols are the shaman's way of distilling the journey and presenting information in a way the community can appreciate. They are not lies, but rather a system used to communicate a little-understood reality.

The SSC represents a discrete altered state of consciousness, following Charles Tart's categorizations.[34] The reality encountered is different from what Tart calls the consensus reality (Castaneda's ordinary reality and Harner's ordinary state of consciousness), but not necessarily to be equated with other kinds of altered states of consciousness, such as those noted in REM or dream sleep, hypnosis, meditation, while in a coma, or after taking psychedelic drugs. Peters and Price-Williams analyzed shamanic practices in forty-two cultures and also concluded that shamanic ecstasy was a specific type of altered state.[35] The notion that there exists only a consensus reality and that every other perception is pathological has significantly impeded the taxonomy of altered states. I submit that the SSC is indeed different from those states cited above, but may correspond to the realm of consciousness described by the mystics, and expounded upon by such fine writers on the topic as Evelyn Underhill and William James, e.g., a state of insight into the depths of truth, unplumbed by the discursive intellect, and used to establish a conscious relation with the Absolute.[36]

The SSC corresponds significantly to Lawrence LeShan's description of "clairvoyant reality," which he uses to describe states of being experienced by both mystics and psychic healers. He contrasts clairvoyant reality with sensory reality, where information comes in through the senses, time is discrete and moves only in one direction, and space serves as a barrier for information exchange. The clairvoyant reality he describes as timeless, where objects may exist but only as part of a unified whole, and neither time nor space can prevent information exchange.[37] His definition, then, is akin to the idea of a nonordinary reality as stated by Castaneda, as well as the SSC. LeShan's in-depth field studies, conducted with a fine scientific eye, enabled him to classify types of psychic healing, replicate it himself in controlled environments, and later to develop a theoretical framework for such events. This is how any scientific pursuit must begin.

LeShan's work is quite relevant to the theme of his book. Although I have not mentioned the word "psychic" specifically, psychic healing, as he describes it, is well within the rubric of the type of healing with the imagination that I have previously categorized as transpersonal healing. It could be argued that mystics and psychic healers are also shamans, since they enter an altered state of consciousness at will to help other persons, use spirit guides, etc. However, the definition of shamanism implies that a social role is being served that is integral to and recognizable by the community.[38] Psychics and mystics normally do not meet the latter qualification. Of a certainty, what LeShan and others refer to as psychic phenomena are aspects of shamanism: clairvoyance, precognition, telepathy, mediumship, special diagnostic and healing abilities. Regardless of terminology, the territory appears to be the same. In this vein, LeShan quotes the visionary Louis Claude de Saint-Martin: "All mystics speak the same language and come from the same country."[39]

The clairvoyant reality, according to LeShan, is reached by means of prayer, or techniques of viewing the healee from a spiritual perspective, or some other technique, such as meditation, which alters the state of consciousness. The healer doesn't try to do anything to the healee; he/she merely tries to unite, merge, become one with him or her. Deep, intense caring or love focused on the healee is described as the heart of the healing mechanism. Both the healer and healee, in a special moment, "know" their integral part in the universe, which places the healee in a different existential position. "He [the healee] was back home in the universe; he was no longer 'cut off' . . . He was completely enfolded and included in the cosmos with his 'being,' his 'uniqueness,' his individuality enhanced."[40] LeShan noted that under these conditions sometimes positive biological changes took place.

The SSC in a Research Perspective

The clairvoyant reality, the SSC, the mystic experience that brings knowledge and insight from sources beyond, can only happen if the barriers separating self from nonself become fluid, and the imagination reaches out beyond the intellect. What is implied here is that the barriers are also a function of the imagination, and can be lifted during specific states of consciousness. In the reports of those who have traveled to these other realities, as we have noted from LeShan and others, it is enough to just "be" there with the expressed purpose of healing in order for healing to occur. Remember, in the shamanic world health is harmony. The transpersonal healer claims to be able to reharmonize or "heal" the patient by readjusting his/her relationship to the rest of the universe, and can do this in an instant of recognizing the divine unity.

How can this be understood within a more scientific framework? The equations and "thought experiments" of quantum physicists, as well as their comments on the behavior of the universe as a metaphor for their observations of subatomic particles, have been employed by LeShan in conjunction with his treatment of clairvoyant reality and the mystical experience, and by Capra to analogize the experience of the mystic, as well as shaman and shamaniclike realities.[41]

Beyond the consensual validation of the phenomenological aspects of the SSC and the quantum analogies, there is scant information on either biochemical or neurophysiological correlates. Dr. Joe Kamiya recently attempted to record physiological data from Michael Harner during a shamanic journey. However, he feels movement artifacts made the data of questionable validity.[42] Most of the standard equipment used to monitor physiological function, particularly brain waves, requires a stationary subject. New developments in telemetric recording devices should be useful in recording and delineating the SSC from other types of altered states.

Two types of data may have relevance for understanding the SSC from the vantage point of basic science. One set of information comes from subjects who have had physiological parameters recorded during what they describe as out-of-the-body (OOB) experiences; the second set comes from studies of the effects of reduced stimulation. The first example is a single, but well-documented, case study by Tart, who recorded brain waves (EEG), galvanic skin response (GSR), and heart rate from a woman who experienced being

OOB frequently during sleep. His results were quite surprising. During what were believed to be the times the OOB state was reported, alpha activity was 1½ cycles per second slower than the subject's normal alpha, and no REMs (rapid eye movements), which normally accompany dreaming, were recorded. Other physiological parameters indicated there was no physiological arousal, despite the reports of heightened mental activity. Tart reported that such a state had never been described in the sleep literature: it could not be classified as any of the known stages of sleep nor was it a Stage 1 (drowsy) pattern, nor was it a waking pattern.[43]

Even though the shamans often describe traveling out of their bodies to strange and exotic places, the OOB states seem to have an air of uncontrollability about them that is unlike the shamanic state of consciousness. Therefore, data on the OOB states may not be truly representative. Information on lucid dreaming, or dreams where conscious control is exerted over the contents and the dreamer is aware of existing simultaneously in the dream as well as the ordinary reality, may be more relevant. The lucid dream is coupled with vivid imagery, a sense of dissociation, and feelings of moving out of the physical body. An ability to dream in this way has been well described by Castaneda and others as being important to shamanic "seeing."[44] Physiological parameters are not yet available, to my knowledge, on this particular phenomena.

Out-of-the-body "journeys" have been reported following significant periods of sensory deprivation, sensory overload, or monotonous or repetitive stimulation—all three of which are part of the ritual for attaining the SSC. One of the most logical experimental paradigms for investigating the SSC, therefore, is a situation of controlled sensory deprivation, or restricted environmental stimulation technique (REST is the acronym chosen by the leading investigators in the area, and will be used here).

The usual experimental milieu involves either a flotation tank or a room with reduced stimulation. The findings from the extensive work in this area, as recently reported in a most thorough and scholarly work by Suedfeld, indicate that the response to reduced or restricted stimulation is culture specific, and it manifests in certain ways and changes over time as anxiety, motivation, and the experiential complex is altered.[45] Most people surely don't participate in REST to attain the SSC, and experiments are rarely conducted to study the effect of REST on self-discovery, or transcendental states. Generalizations from REST to the SSC must be made with this caution in mind.

In the flotation tank, particularly, the logical bounds between self and nonself are quickly dissolved. The body is free floating, nonconstricted by clothing; sensory and motor systems are not called into play; and there is no competition for the energy required by the imagination. The brain is allowed space and time to range freely through areas that are beyond sensory input and motor exposition. There is widespread agreement among researchers that under such conditions creativity and special problem-solving abilities are enhanced, and vivid visual images are commonly reported as the source of new information.

In some of the earliest work in the area of deprivation, Heron and Zubek, Welch, and Saunders, reported unusual shifts into slower alpha activity following 96 hours and 14 days, respectively, of perceptual deprivation, corresponding to Tart's findings on the OOB experience.[46] Suedfeld, in reviewing the findings on EEG and REST, offers support for this effect on alpha activity, and cites evidence pointing to its persistence days after exposure to the REST situation.[47] An increase in theta waves (the very slow brain waves associated with creativity) is noted, particularly in the temporal region of the brain, but not with the same consistency as the change in alpha waves. Therefore, it appears that a slowing of alpha might be of relevance in discriminating aspects of the SSC, but the significance of the relationship remains unclear.

The role of reduced stimulation in facilitating altered states of consciousness has not been well studied, even though shifts in consciousness, out-of-body phenomena, and transcendent experiences are frequently reported by the subjects involved in the research.[48] That they are not the subject of research itself is not surprising, given the extant scientific prohibition on studying anything but the consensual reality. John Lilly's work, of course, is a notable exception, as he has explored the depths of his own consciousness during flotation, and analyzed it with his own mixture of scientific and mystical points of view.[49]

The imagery associated with REST has been reviewed by Zuckerman, who concludes that the phenomena are primarily visual (as opposed to auditory, as would be true of hallucinations), and move from simple to complex as the length of time in the REST situation increases.[50] Suedfeld reviews a work by G. F. Reed (in press), who described the increased involuntary imagery, particularly visual imagery associated with REST, as a corollary to the decrease in logical, analytical thought that is based upon verbal symbols. Further, he hypothesizes that stimulus deprivation increases the prevalence of intuitive, configurational procedures (the type of information processing that has come, rightly or not, to characterize the right hemisphere of the brain's cerebral cortex), at the expense of analysis, language, and logic (the putated activities of the left hemisphere). REST is suggested as an "environmental way to achieve temporary dominance of right hemisphere functioning . . . and may be an externally structured analogue of meditation and similar states."[51]

Shamanism and Schizophrenia

There is a persistent debate among scholars on whether or not shamanism is a culturally sanctioned vocation for the mentally deranged, in particular schizophrenics. Although this position was a leading anthropological point of view until the 1940s,[52] it has a few contemporary advocates as well. Among those most frequently cited are Devereux, who steadfastly maintains there is no excuse for not regarding the shamans as neurotic or even psychotic, and Silverman, who likens the SSC to acute schizophrenia.[53] On the other hand, Jilek feels the pathology label to be "absolutely untenable"[54] after his years of experience with shamans in North America, Africa, Haiti, South America, Thailand and New Guinea. He is trained in both psychiatry and anthropology, and believes the pathology position will become increasingly refuted as the field of cross-cultural psychiatry is expanded.

A recent definitive article by Richard Noll marshals the evidence on both sides of the controversy, and concludes that the schizophrenic metaphor results from a failure to discriminate between the phenomenological differences of the SSC and the schizophrenic state of consciousness.[55] He cites the most important distinction as one of volition: The shaman as "master of ecstasy"[56] willfully enters and leaves the altered state; the schizophrenic exerts no control over such activity and is the hapless victim of delusion, with a notable impairment in role functioning. Harner emphasizes the necessity for the shaman to function in a commendable manner in ordinary reality, as well as in the SSC, in order to be believable and to maintain status within the community.[57] Separating out the contents of different levels of reality is impossible for the schizophrenic, but, as Noll states, "the validity of both realms is acknowledged by the shaman, whose mastery derives from his ability to not confuse the two."[58]

Without dwelling at undue length upon this subject—one would hope it would die a natural death from lack of evidence supporting the schizophrenic position—I would like to mention two relevant issues. First is a reiteration that the problem in identifying the role and person of the shaman, as well as the mystic, stems from the Western psychological categorization of all behaviors not within the "norm" (or common to the majority), as deviant in the negative sense. Traditional psychology has no theoretical umbrella to cover the "supernormal"—the creative genius, the highly imaginative, the person who enters altered states of consciousness at will—except to classify that individual as mentally ill, or a hair's breadth from it. Newer theories of personality development propounded by Ken Wilber and Elmer and Alyce Green, and the visions of psychology proposed by James Hillman, all include the notion that "normal" is by no means the most evolved possibility.[59]

The second point is that there has been a tendency on the part of some observers to elevate the traditional status of schizophrenia,[60] as well as epilepsy,[61] regarding them as potentiators of tremendous psychological breakthrough and insight, not unlike those reported by the mystics. The ancient and widely scattered practice of endowing epileptics with a favored position within the ranks of shamanism, the observations that shamanic ecstasy resembles a kind of controlled seizure activity, and the acute mental and physical anguish associated with the initiation or "divine call" of the shaman[62] do need to be explored in this regard.

The persons diagnosed with schizophrenia and some forms of epilepsy both have in common exceptionally high amounts of mental activity. In some kinds of epilepsy, the epileptic patient's EEG is characterized by bursts of persistent brain activity, localized at first, then expanding, recruiting a wake of other neurons, until there is an electrical explosion which results in a full-blown seizure, followed by a comatose state. Auras, hallucinations, massive motor activity, bizarre sensory phenomena are all possible. The schizophrenic, too, is confronted with an onslaught of imagery—so much so that figure is not well separated from ground and the inner world becomes an active, incoherent buzz. Inner experience and facts received through the senses are not well discriminated. Because of the rampage of neuronal firing, it is possible that both the schizophrenic and epileptic patients could experience all that consciousness has to offer, from the most primitive, preverbal images to glimpses of the transcendent landscapes reported by the shamans and mystics.

As Wilber has stated with regard to the schizophrenic, "The disruption of the editing and filtering functions of egoic translation (secondary process, reality principle, syntaxical structuring, etc.) leaves the individual open to and unprotected from *both the lower and the higher* levels of consciousness." And in discriminating the mystical state from the phenomenology of the schizophrenic, he allows that the mystic is exploring and mastering some of the same higher realms that overpower the schizophrenic. In contrast, "The mystic *seeks* progressive evolution. He trains for it. It takes most of a lifetime—with luck—to reach permanent, mature, transcendent and unity structures." He also says "Mysticism is not regression in service of the ego, but evolution in transcendence of the ego."[63] His statements would certainly be agreed upon as representing the shamans by the contemporary scholars who view an evolved state of consciousness as a prerequisite for the vocation.

So, with the shamans' sanity tentatively documented, whether or not it is broadly applicable to all who call themselves shamans, let us move on to the more specific behaviors that are given credit for calling forth the healing powers of the imagination.

Setting the Stage: Rituals and Symbols

Shamanic rituals and symbols provide one of the more fascinating sagas of how human beings attempt to relate to the supernatural in order to create a condition of health, in its broadest sense. My purpose, though, is not to offer a compendium of shamanic practice, since that has been done quite well already by authors whose names are sprinkled throughout this chapter. I shall only attempt to summarize and offer a few examples.

Four issues can be abstracted out of the voluminous writings on shamanistic ritual and practice. The first, and one that cannot be overemphasized, was discussed in the previous section: The rituals and symbols of healing have a quite different, yet very real, meaning in the nonordinary reality or shamanic state of consciousness. Second, many rituals and symbols are culturally determined, and speak to the needs of only a special population. Next, there are some similar symbols and rituals found in all parts of the world, indicating a kind of collective unconscious at work. And finally, and most important for the thesis of this book, while these tools of the trade can't in any way be separated or omitted from the concept of shamanism, it is not the tools and rituals that heal, it is the power endowed in them by the imagination.

First of all, I will discuss the ubiquitous shamanistic practices.

Rituals to Enter the Shamanic State of Consciousness

Since shamans do their healing work in something other than the wide-awake, beta brain wave, linear-thought state of mind, they naturally first have to adopt satisfactory ways of exiting from that condition. This constitutes the serious beginning of the healing ritual, although the ritual setting itself may have taken days to prepare. Virtually anything that has ever been used to achieve an altered state of consciousness has probably been included in one or another shaman's rituals, with most of the techniques geared toward hypostimulation or hyperstimulation of various sensory systems. Some examples include:

1. *Intensive temperature conditions.* The sweat lodge or saunalike structure is a commonly used vehicle for inducing an altered state of consciousness. A typical lodge might consist of a willow frame, covered with a tarp or some other heavy material to capture the heat. Rocks are heated for hours in a hot fire, and at the time of the sweat, they are placed in the center of the lodge. Usually, there is a prescribed format for entering and leaving the sweat, and for songs and chants of supplication, thanksgiving, and affirmation of the connectedness of all material and nonmaterial aspects of the universe. The heat is periodically intensified by throwing water on the hot stones, and herbs such as sweet grass or sage might be burnt for their special aromas and sacred significance.

A sweat lodge without ritual is just hot; but even with ritual, it can induce a massive systemic effect that includes rapidly increased pulse rate, nausea, dizziness, and syncope (fainting)—in short, the warning signs of the impending medical condition we call heat stroke. I have, on occasion, been more focused upon surviving the ordeal and keeping the inhaled blasts of fiery air from searing their course right through my nostrils, lungs, and beyond, than on having visions. The Indians don't share my concern about the possible ill effects of the procedure, and often prescribe it as a cure for serious illness, even in the young and the elderly. The sauna ritual has a firm European foundation, too, and the Scandinavians have used it for centuries to promote body/mind health. There is little question that the physiological response to such intense stimulation is partially a function of learning set.

From a physical standpoint, there is a biochemical component of high body temperatures during fevers that reflects the natural reaction to toxins, and is correlated to the immune system in action. The artificially induced high temperatures of the sauna may mimic or induce this activity (as does sustained aerobic exercise). Furthermore, the sweat or sauna may act as a sterilization procedure, killing bacteria, viruses and other organisms that thrive at body temperature, but are susceptible to heat. The growth of tumors may also be inhibited when core body temperature is significantly elevated. Heat directed at the tumors has been an experimental treatment for cancer in approximately fifty medical centers in this country. Dr. Seymour Levitt, chief of therapeutic radiology at University Hospital in Minneapolis, has perfected the treatment somewhat by using a Japanese-made heat source that deeply penetrates the skin and heats the tumor to 100° F. Apparently, the heat is not only effective in killing cancer cells, but also makes the surviving cancer cells more vulnerable to radiation and chemotherapy. In any case, drinking lots of water and then taking a sauna results in feelings of detoxification and clearing of the mind. The heat itself can help create an altered state of consciousness and promote the intense concentration necessary for healing.

In addition to such external aids as the sauna or sweat lodge, the ability to self-generate internal heat is typically regarded as necessary for shamanistic healing. One of the putative derivations of the word *shaman* is the Vedic *sram*, "to heat oneself or practice austerities." [64] According to an Eskimo shaman, "Every real shaman has to feel an illumination in his body, in the inside of his head or in his brain, something that gleams like fire, that gives him the power to see with closed eyes into the darkness, into the hidden things or into the future, or into the secrets of another man." [65] Agreement for this premise comes from Evans-Wentz' well-known work on the Tibetan yogins, who, according to Eliade's writings, claim many of the same abilities as the shaman. [66] The advanced yogins are said to be able to produce psychic heat that renders them impervious to temperature extremes, even to long-term exposure to snow while wrapped only in sheets dipped in icy water. [67]

In order to create their special state, the yogins use a process of imagery, one that involves visualizing a sun in various parts of their bodies and the world being permeated by fire. It is said that, as a result of practicing these exercises over a long period of time, the yogin has the ability to learn of past, present and future events.

The relationship between the hypermetabolic state produced by increased heat and the acquisition of unusual knowledge is beyond any scientific interpretation. But consider the incredible mental control over physiology that must be exercised in order for dramatic temperature shifts to be made. Temperature regulation is one of the most complex autonomic functions in the human body. The mere maintenance of homeostatic temperature requires a moment-by-moment interplay between air temperature, skin temperature, and a regulating center in the preoptic hypothalamus in the brain. Such regulation is required even when sitting nude in a comfortable room, since about 12% of body heat is quickly lost under these conditions.

In order to sustain body heat in unusual climes such as the icy Himalayas, or to increase body heat significantly above normal levels as is reported by the shamans, the body has available only three known mechanisms. These are: shivering or other muscular activity; excitation of the chemicals that increase the levels of circulating norepinephrine and epinephrine, and subsequently cellular metabolism; and increased thyroxine output, which also increases the rate of cellular metabolism.[68]

External temperature can be raised by diverting internal body heat to the periphery through an increased rate of blood flow in the skin. As is profusely documented throughout the biofeedback literature, this can be accomplished with various mental techniques such as imagery and relaxation, as well as temperature biofeedback. These procedures have been used effectively to treat a myriad of health conditions, including migraine, Raynaud's Syndrome and other circulatory disorders, arthritis, pain, and stress-related diseases.[69] Increased peripheral temperatures are an indicator of reduced sympathetic nervous system activity, and hence, of a reduced stress response. Of course, none of this may be of any relevance to the Tibetan yogin, nor to the Arctic shamans who also endure extreme cold, since diversion of blood to the periphery would quickly result in a fatal decrease in core temperature. The yogins and shamans have apparently found a means to continue an indefinite heat exchange, which means they have the ability to regenerate those chemicals involved, for a long time. We can only conclude that a powerful ability to self-regulate the thermal response is apparent, and note additionally that those who involve themselves in such affairs regard the internal heat as a pathway to knowledge.

2. *Physical or sensory deprivation.* Physical deprivation takes many forms, and the mystical experience it induces is by no means unique to the shamanistic cultures. It is unfortunate, I suppose, for those of us who live in nondeprived circumstances, that such physical comfort does not breed mysticism. On the other hand,

the mind's enhanced power to create visions in circumstances of deprivation was often regarded as the sole factor that made Nazi concentration camp life tolerable. "The dreams," the survivors say, "those wonderful dreams."

Typically, the shamans fast before doing difficult work. The fast may include dispensing with food, or salt, or even water. Other deprivations include going without sleep for several nights, which may happen anyway in the process of a lengthy ritual. The European shamans, the witches, were accused of eating only beets, roots, and berries (i.e., avoiding animal protein and milk products) to aid them on their shamanic journeying. The Huichol shamans traditionally fasted during their twenty-day trek to the land of the peyote, their place of power. In some cultures the healee may also be advised to abstain from food for a period of days.

Abstinence from sex is universally used to alter the realms of consciousness. This vital life energy is redirected toward healing, or to produce states of bliss (as in the Eastern practice of kundalini). The novice Jívaro shaman, for instance, must abstain from sex for at least five months to gain enough power to cure, and for a whole year in order to become really effective.[70] In Christianity, however, celibacy has quite different origins in that it was believed to protect the holy fathers from the remnants of original sin, and thereby increase their divinity.

The shamanic state of mind is enhanced during instances of sensory deprivation, as well as physical deprivation. Most ceremonial work is done in the darkness, or with the eyes covered to shut out ordinary reality. Visions are sought by staying isolated in deep caves, or in the monotonous landscape of the tundra or desert. Nordland has noted that sensory deprivation studies (reviewed briefly in an earlier section of this chapter) may provide insights on shamanism. "It appears to be clear that monotony is the basis of many forms of shamanism: monotonous song, drumming, music, dance with rhythmic movements. At other times it can be the restriction of movement, staring into the flames, darkness, even masks with special effects for the eyes."[71]

In sum, the shamans use a variety of culturally sanctioned means of deprivation to find their way into the SSC. Their methods have the potential to cause significant physical and mental shifts by inducing electrolyte imbalances, hypoglycemia, dehydration, sleeplessness, and loss of sensory input. In short, they seem willing to push their bodies to the physiological limits in order to awaken the mind. What the modern world regards as dangerous threats to health, even to life itself, are viewed by the shaman as routes to knowledge.

3. *The use of sacred plants.* Hallucinogenic substances are employed throughout shamanic healing traditions as the fastest way to encounter the supernatural; however, it is important to realize that the plants are not essential to shamanic work. Prem Das, a young man trained in both Yogic and Huichol traditions, views the sacred plants as an intermediate step only, and says that advanced practitioners no longer have need of them. The topic has captured the imagination of anthropologists since the 1960s, when there was a great heightening of awareness of drugs in this country. The voluminous reading available includes the following: The role of hallucinogens in some North and South American and European shamanic traditions has been reviewed in a book edited by Harner; Gordon Wasson has reviewed the use of the fly-agaric mushroom amongst the Siberians, East Indians, and Scandinavians; Weston LaBarre has written a classic treatise on peyote; and Peter Furst has edited a volume on the ritual use of hallucinogens.[72]

Anthropologist Carlos Castaneda, too, has described in widely-read detail his use of psychotropic power plants as visionary aides while under the mentorship of Yaqui shaman, Don Juan. There are mixed reactions in scientific circles regarding the authenticity and meaning of Castaneda's experiences, but there is some consensus that even if they were confabulated, they are highly representative of cross-cultural encounters with the supernatural.[73]

The greater number of Castaneda's experiences are not properly within the shamanic healing tradition, but should best be classified as sorcery, or power seeking. However, his journeying to find the place "between the worlds" involves using techniques of the imagination identical to those of healing shamans. Don Juan guided Castaneda through episodes following the use of datura (or Jimson weed); Psilocybe, a mushroom species; and peyote. But the drugs were resorted to only after it became obvious that Castaneda's waking state of consciousness was too restricted to expand into the mystical, magical nonordinary reality. Castaneda stated that he would always question the validity of his experiences under the influence of the psychotropic plants, and he regarded the final stage of consciousness expansion—the pure wondering perception of viewing the world without interpretation—as not possible with the drugs.[74]

On the other hand, since there is a relationship between the shamanic tradition and the use of sacred plants, we do need to consider their use, and certainly what relationship they might play in a shamanistic renaissance. First of all, as mentioned, they provide a rapid means of altering consciousness. Second, in preliterate societies, both death and dreams foretold of other states of being, and the answers to these, the greatest of mysteries, were most likely sought through experience, and not intellectual discourse. The noted psychotropic effects of the power plants, such as losing the boundaries of self, enhanced awareness of the continuity of all things, and a sense of awe and wonder, gave the shamans the insight and knowledge they craved of the world beyond the senses. Because of these properties, the plants are universally called "medicine" and referred to as being "sacred." Using them for recreational purposes would be unthinkable.

Unlike those of some mystical persuasions, the shamans do not seek the enlightenment for its sake alone, but with the explicit purpose of aiding the community. Their path is circular; i.e., they move up and out into other realms, but then they return again with knowledge and power. Whenever the sacred plants are used in the healing arts, their effects must be subtle enough to permit the shaman to function in this way. Ritual work can't be done in a comatose state of oblivion, or when control is relinquished to narcotic effects. The shamans ingest appropriate amounts of the plants to allow for postexperience recall, and enough awareness for them to be cognizant of the multiple realities they are encountering. One foot, so to speak, stays in ordinary reality.

Nature has provided an abundant supply of this medicine, especially in the Americas. Particularly ubiquitous in South and Central America is the use of the Banisteriopsis vine (often called *yagé* or *ayahuasca*). The visionary process used among the Sharanahua Indians of eastern Peru is particularly interesting from a standpoint of the ability of the imagination to diagnose as well as cure. The shaman will ask seriously ill patients to describe their symptoms and their dreams. The patients normally report images that coincide with categories of curing songs the shaman has learned during the extended apprenticeship. (The singing and chanting is an important accoutrement to the *ayahuasca*, since without the words, only visions of snakes are supposed to appear.) The dream images that are reported are usually simple: the sun, a bird, someone climbing a mountain.[75]

Early in the evening of the healing ceremony, the shaman and other men of the tribe drink the *ayahuasca*; the men chant, the shaman sings the appropriate song, and a vision appears of the image from the patient's dream. With great, intense clarity, the shaman describes this vision. Siskind says: "The sharing of symbols between at least two people is the basis for any communication system. Dream and vision symbolism among the Sharanahua does not involve a one-to-one relationship of meaning and symbol, but neither is there complete free rein for idiosyncratic dreaming or hallucinating. Both shaman and patient are bound by the limits of the curing song classification of symbol and symptoms." The selection of symbols must coincide with the symbol system common to the culture. "Yet, there is sufficient overlap and redundancy of symbols, especially with regard to the most common serious ailments, bloody diarrhea, stomach-ache, and grippe with high fever, for individual feelings to be expressed by the patient and picked up by the shaman."[76]

The use of peyote, too, is an ever expanding tradition in the New World, and is believed to open up the skylights of consciousness. "There is a doorway within our minds that usually remains hidden and secret until the time of death. The Huichol word for it is *nieríka*. Nieríka is a cosmic portway or interface between so-called ordinary and nonordinary realities. It is a passageway and at the same time a barrier between worlds."[77]

The Huichol use cactus gathered from the Sacred Land of the Peyote to facilitate entry into the nieríka. According to Prem Das, the Huichol shamanistic tradition tends to have more of a transpersonal nature, while The Native American Church, a remarkable confederation of several Indian tribes, uses peyote as part of a Christian, humanistic ceremonial.[78] (The Native American Church, founded in Mexico some 150 years ago, has been elaborated particularly by the Kiowa tribes in this country. The members chose to focus on the problems of living in today's world as opposed to the shamanic journeying.)

Forms of the datura plant and mushrooms with hallucinogenic properties are frequently used by both American and Old World shamans. The mushroom has been especially provocative to anthropologists and nonanthropologists alike, who have stalked the legendary soma and identified it with the fly-agaric mushrooms of Europe and Asia,[79] and supped on the Flesh of Gods, the widely used Psilocybe mushrooms of Mexico.[80] "The Mazatecs say that the mushrooms speak. If you ask a shaman where his imagery comes from, he is likely to reply: I didn't say it, the mushrooms did. . . . The shamans who eat them, their function is to speak, they are the speakers who chant and sing the truth, they are the oral poets of their people, the doctors of the word, they who tell what is wrong and how to remedy it, the seers and oracles, the ones possessed by the voice."[81]

Part of a Mazatec song of the medicine woman goes as follows: "Woman of medicines and curer, who walks with her appearance and her soul . . . she is the woman of the remedy and the medicine. She is the woman who speaks. The woman who puts everything together. Doctor woman. Woman of words. Wise woman of problems."[82] So she sings, talking of a communal world, searching for the tracks of meaning, healing in the wake of the chemical transformation wrought by the magic mushroom.

In Europe, the witches, who both Harner and Eliade identify as being involved in shamanic practices, also transformed their state of awareness with hallucinogenic substances.[83] There, nature's bounty provided a psychedelic selection with considerably more impact than the gentle mushrooms of the Mazatec medicine woman. The deadly nightshade (belladonna), mandrake root, henbane, and datura were combined by various recipes into a "flying oyl," and on "certain days or nights they anoint a staff and ride on it to the appointed place or anoint themselves under the arms and in other hairy places.[84]

The high atropine content of the European shaman's pharmacopeia assured ready absorption through the skin, particularly the sensitive vaginal tissue. A broomstick, thusly anointed, became the steed for shamanic journeys, and the dangerous drug road often led to several days of oblivion, followed by amnesia. For this reason, Harner does not believe the witches used the plants in healing ritual, but only to make contact with the supernatural.[85]

We must evaluate the "sacred plant" aspect of healing cautiously. The modern world of medicine would give a collective shudder at the thought of the healer taking powerful dangerous chemicals, especially when the same states of mind can be achieved through nonchemical means. But is there not a parallel here between this and providing the *patient* with powerful dangerous chemicals, when evidence is rapidly accumulating that the imagination, itself, can create every conceivable physical change? The chemical crutches, in both instances, are only evolutionary steps in learning to use the forces of consciousness to heal.

I would like to make one final observation on this theme: When the supernatural path is circular, as in the case of shamans who move into those realms and return to do the healing work of the world, those who travel that path bring back something of the glory of their visualizations. The beautiful sacred art of the shamanic cultures is precisely that. The yarn pictures, the beadwork, and the sandpaintings are all attempts to share the spirit realm through the media of this world. The visionary experiences were also preserved in the shaman's medicine bundle: feathers, beads, skeletons of animals, stones, shells, dried plants, even the European "junk" found its way into the North American Indians' sacred bundles. Sometimes the objects represent special gifts given to the shaman in the SSC. Grossinger makes the point that the attachment for trinkets, which white man has never truly appreciated, comes from the symbolic vestment of the visionary experience. "Several generations after the vision, the medicine bundle is an objective technique of sorts. It has songs, herbs, charms, stories, all keyed to the original revelation and added to by those who have used the medicine."[86]

Recently I happened to enter an old house, built in the 1920s by an anthropologist who had immersed himself in Indian studies. The house was constructed of handmade adobe, built around large semicircular fireplaces, in the style of the Indians who populated that region years before. As I entered the room containing the bathtub, which was the sole modern convenience in the house, I experienced a queasy feeling that something unbalanced had happened here. A hippie commune had left the mark of its tenure forever preserved in hundreds of small rough tiles that covered the inner surface of the tub. The chaotic, bright, designs had the same eery aspect as the day-glo art of the sixties: mixed religious symbolism and colors foreign to nature, even ugly in this ordinary reality. It had "bad vibes," as they said then. "Ah," said I, as I recognized it as the drug cult's version of sacred art, an attempt to move along the circular path and bring back the outer reaches to the linear mind. It spoke to me of the tenants' attempts to use the drugs as medicine; yet not having a map to guide the way, they were able to represent only the cacophony of an unfiltered consciousness.

The drugs as they were used in a spiritual tradition were medicine, the best medicine the world knew for thousands of years. But for a culture that has progressively alienated itself from the spirit world in all its institutions, a culture that has tried its hardest to separate mind from body, the drugs provide only a tantalizing taste of mysticism, which our cultural myth cannot explain and will not incorporate.

    4. Auditory aides to altered states. Repeated, monotonous stimulation of any sense changes the focus of awareness. For the shaman, the usual choice of sound stimulus comes from drums, rattles, sticks, or other percussion instruments. Other sounds, such as the high-pitched whirring produced by the whistling vessels found in Peru and Central America, may also have been used in shamanic work.[87] Chants and songs, of course, are important to healing ceremonies of all cultures.

Normally, the chants are phonemes strung together. There is no ready interpretation or translation for them available in the language of ordinary reality, only in feeling states. They may serve the purpose of bypassing the logical, language part of our brains, and touching the intuitive. (A devout Catholic friend made the observation that Mass lost much of its impact when it was no longer given in Latin. "When you didn't know what the words meant, you communicated more directly with God.")

The chants might have come to the shamans' awareness during the solitude of the vision quest, or been gifted to them by a passing eagle, or heard in a dream. Or they may be traditional healing or power chants, with the original source unknown. The chants have a pulsating rhythm that, like the drum beats, synchronizes the body function and movements. Shamans may also use songs with distinctive meaning. The songs of the Navaho shaman, for instance, are so incredibly complicated that one writer has likened them to the equivalent of a complete recitation of the New Testament by heart.[88] Most often, the songs are disease chasers, not entrees into the shamanic state of consciousness.

The shaman's drum reigns as the most important means to enter other realities, and as one of the most universal characteristics of shamanism. The drum can be made of just about anything that sets up a reasonably deep tone. According to Drury, it is made of the wood of the world tree, and the skin is sometimes directly linked to the animal the shaman uses to encounter the place of spirit.[89] The wonderfully resonant water drums may be made of old metal cooking pots filled partway with water and wrapped with an animal skin—a time-consuming process that must be repeated often during long ceremonials.[90]

The sounds of the percussion instruments and the rattles are time-honored methods for consciousness altering, and are considered to have a numbing or analgesic effect. "On a contemplative level," says Drury, "The sound of the drum thus acts as a focusing device for the shaman. It creates an atmosphere of concentration and resolve, enabling him to sink deep into trance as he shifts his atten-

tion to the inner journey of the spirit."[91] Several physiological facts
support the role of sound in this regard. First, the auditory tracts
pass directly into the reticular activating system (RAS) of the brain
stem. The RAS is a massive "nerve net" and functions to coordinate
sensory input and motor tone, and to alert the cortex to incoming
information. Sound, traveling on these pathways, is capable of activating the entire brain.[92] Strong, repetitive neuronal firing in the
auditory pathways and ultimately in the cerebral cortex, such as
would be experienced from the drums, could theoretically compete
successfully for cognitive awareness. Other sensory stimuli from
ordinary reality, including pain, could thus be gated or filtered out.
The mind would then be free to expand into other realms.

The pain model established by Melzack and Wall (i.e., gate
theory) can be appropriately applied here. Their model is the most
widely cited, universally accepted model of the pain mechanism.
(With the recent advances in identifying pain-modulating chemicals
such as the endorphins, the gate theory is considered only part of
the story, however.) Melzack and Wall have proposed that since the
pain message travels on small, sluggish fibers, the perception of
pain can be effectively blocked by other incoming stimuli traveling
on more rapid conducting fibers.[93] The model has been used to account for the pain-relieving effects of acupuncture, mild trans-
cutaneous electrical stimulation, and massage. Powerful sounds,
such as the drumming, which have the capacity to activate all brain
centers, could well fulfill the requirement for faster, more competi-
tive stimulation.

In a study with severely burned babies, I used sounds of a heart
beat recorded in utero—highly similar in nature to the drum beats—
to create anesthesia. The heart sounds were capable of inducing
sleep even during painful dressing changes. After the children became accustomed to the tape recorder in their cribs, they would fall
asleep within minutes after it was turned on. The seventy-two beats
per minute of the average heart is much slower than theta, but it is
possible the sounds could have stimulated delta brain wave patterns
which range between .5 to 4.0 cycles per second. There was no question, at any rate, that it served as an effective sensory block, whatever the mechanism involved.

The direct effect of acoustic stimulation on the brain was reported in a classic study by Neher. He recorded EEG's in normal
subjects while they listened to low frequency, high amplitude sound
from a drum. The purpose of the study was to determine whether

the drumming could cause "auditory driving," so named because some stimuli are known to "drive" or provoke a pattern of firing frequencies in surrounding systems.[94]

In Neher's work, auditory driving responses were elicited at three, four, six, and eight beats per second, and the subjects expressed subjective accounts of both visual and auditory imagery. He concluded that susceptibility to rhythmic stimulation is enhanced by stress and metabolic imbalances (hypoglycemia, fatigue, etc.; all to be expected as part of the shamanic ritual). He also proposed that sound stimulation in the frequency range of four to seven cycles per second would be most effective in ceremonial work, since this could enhance the theta rhythms that occur in the temporal auditory regions of the cortex. Theta rhythms, I might add, have also been shown to be related to creativity, unusual problem-solving, vivid imagery, and states of reverie.[95] Unfortunately, while Neher's premise is sound, his study was critically flawed because he did not control for movement artifact. The EEG cannot discriminate between eye blinks, head nods, and brain waves, and what Neher may have been recording was any or all of these, done in keeping time with the drum's rhythm.

Jilek offers still more information on the theta driving capacity of drumming in work with the Salish Indians during their spirit dance ceremonial. In analyzing the records of drumming, he determined the rhythms encompassed a frequency range of from .8 to 5.0 cycles per second. One-third of the frequencies were above 3.0 cycles per second, or quite close to the theta wave frequency. He also notes that the rhythmic acoustic stimulation in the ceremonies involves many drums and is significantly more intensive than Neher used in his experiments.[96]

Let us consider now the mechanism through which auditory stimuli might serve to alter brain function. A neuron carrying information through the sensory complex of the nervous system can either fire or not fire, and messages in all systems are based upon the frequency of this firing, as will be discussed in detail in Chapter 4. For example, suppose sensory information from some system was able to "drive" the entire motor cortex. Then the rate of neuronal firing in the motor cortex would be identical with whatever frequency was occurring in the driving sensory system. This could produce extremely bizarre and maladaptive effects if it happened readily, which it apparently does not except in severe epileptics. Most of the work on "driving" has been done with the visual system. In studies conducted with animals, persons with epilepsy and normal subjects, a repetitive visual stimulus such as a strobe light has been shown to cause "photic driving" in widespread areas of the cortex.[97]

There is evidence that the brain activity driven by the original stimulus can continue long after the stimulation has ceased, and the continued neural discharge may be responded to behaviorally as if the light were still flashing.[98] What appear to be hallucinated experiences actually have a neurological component in the visual system. In view of these findings, there is reason to believe the auditory system, put to the proper test, would have similar potency in controlling cortical function. (The visual studies also offer a neurological basis for altering state of consciousness by staring into the fire or at candles during rituals.)

Evidence from meditation research indicates the auditory stimulus need not be external, but only imaged, in order to effect a significant physiological change.[99] Transcendental meditation, the relaxation response (espoused by Herbert Benson), and other adaptations of *raja yoga* involve imaging a word or sound (or mantra) over and over again. One might call this an imaged chant. Physiological response and benefits have been reported to include decreases in heart rate, blood pressure and muscle tension, and increased alpha and theta activity in the EEG. The methods have been touted as an important method of controlling stress and establishing a "wakeful hypometabolic state,"[100] which can restore the body to a comfortable, healthful level of homeostatic balance.

5. *Spirit allies.* The last aspect of the imagination that we will deal with here is one of the outstanding characteristics of shamanhood: the spirit helpers. These are the spirit forms, usually of animals, who protect the shaman in dangerous work, and whom they claim as the source of their knowledge. These are the professors in that medical school of the great beyond. For the Japanese shaman, they may take the exalted form of a transformation of the Buddha.[101] A Netsilik Eskimo, regarded as a major shaman of his time, had no fewer than seven spirits—a sea scorpion, a killer whale, a black dog with no ears, and ghosts of three dead people.[102] In American Indian tribes, the spirits may be animals having special cultural significance—bears, eagles, wolves.

Deer are widely associated with shamanic work. In Siberia, real-life reindeer shared the fly-agaric journeys with the shaman.[103] In Iran and China, deer horns are still valued as both magic and medicine,[104] and powdered horn is widely sold as an aphrodisiac. The deer spirit is believed to leave the sacred peyote buttons as tracks to guide the shamans on their supernatural course, according to the myths of the Huichols. Even in prehistoric times, as mentioned earlier, it seems that the deer had healing significance, based on man/deer shaman art forms that have been identified as dating from the beginning of recorded history.

In Europe, the power animals of the witches, who are believed to have been practicing aspects of shamanic healing, were greatly feared. In a volume printed in 1618 entitled *The County Justice* by Michal Dalton, Gentleman of Lincoln, two of the seven methods of discovery of witches he cited related to their relationship with their animals: "They have ordinarily a familiar or spirit which appeareth to them" and "The said familiar hath some bigg or place upon their body where he sucketh them."[105] Owning a pet cast immediate suspicion upon a woman; and during the reign of Louis XV of France, sacks of condemned cats were burned on the public square where witches were tortured. There has been some speculation that the fury of the plagues was increased by this mass destruction of the infested rats' natural enemy.

The spirit allies need not always be animals—sometimes the spirits metamorphose into human form. An early report of an Indian aboriginal shaman of the Savara tribe describes a guide taking the form of a girl who dictated who the shaman should marry in ordinary reality, and gave her instructions on how to care for her husband. The guide, herself, bore the shaman two children whom she later carried to the underworld.[106]

Healers may have as their guides people who actually lived on earth at one time. Krippner and Villoldo, in their book *Realms of Healing*, tell of Dona Pachita, a Mexican "psychic surgeon" whose spirit guide is Cuahutemoc, the last great Aztec prince, and of Arigo, a Brazilian healer whose guide is "Dr. Fritz," a German physician whom he has seen in visions since his youth.[107] It could be argued whether these two fall within a true definition of shamanism, yet the point is made that imaginary guides are often used in the practice of traditional healing.

While circumstances vary, it is usually believed that the spirits are always lurking around, but may go unrecognized by their earthly charges. The shaman not only has exceptionally powerful allies, but the ability to stay in communication with them, which differentiates the shaman from laypersons who may also have spirit helpers. The shaman is chosen by the spirits after a period of turmoil, which, depending upon one's point of view, could be classified as "an acute psychological crisis, a true mystical religious experience, a physical illness, or a psychosis."[108]

"Spirit possession," as described in the anthropological literature on shamanism, should be carefully distinguished from demonic possession. The spirits do not induce the shaman to perform evil acts, but are instead teachers. The periods of discomfort when the spirits are said to "take possession" are intended to be necessary learning experiences for the healing vocation. Noll, in reviewing the opinion on this matter, concludes that "Much of what is summarily labeled as 'possession' by trained observers may be a willful visionary experience for the shaman."[109]

Now, it is possible to analyze the use of spirit guides with the tools of science, and derive perfectly sane and acceptable reasons for any truths that might evolve from spirit communication. If the spirits only symbolize the intuitive, then communication would be akin to the left side of the brain asking the right side, "What's happening?" The shamans would be those individuals who could best combine logic and intuition. However, in shamanism humans are naturally in communication with animals, spirits, and even rocks, because they are one and the same in the great unified order of things. Shamans are those who can acutely sense and move with the fabric of the universes, and who are led along their healing path by sources of wisdom manifest in what have come to be known as spirit guides. Again, the shamans' qualifications are undeniably based upon their demonstration of a vivid imagination, and their ability to stay in control of the situation—regardless of where their information comes from.

Specific Cultural Practices

The shaman's practice is highly integrated with the belief system of the culture, and he/she must have the skill to create an atmosphere replete with trust, credibility, and enough creativity and outrageousness to let the patient know that something powerful is about to happen.

The Yakut shamans of Siberia wear cloaks of jingling metal; they chant, beat their drums, and when emotions build to a high pitch, they try to frighten the spirit out with terrifying gestures. In Africa, the shamans create a straw image of a pig, and go through a ceremony of removing the illness from the patient and shipping it off into the pig. Then, the animal is placed on a road so that a passerby who kicks it will absorb the disease.[110]

For extremely serious healing, such as in the case of soul loss, the Puget Sound or West Coast Salish Indians use a spirit canoe ritual. Anywhere from six to twelve shamans are hired, and imaginary canoes are formed as they stand in parallel rows. Every shaman has a pole or paddle to push the canoe, and beside each of them lies their magic cedar board, covered with visionary art of their first spirit canoe adventure. With the auditory accompaniment of rattles, drums and chants, the shamans' spirits sink through the earth, each singing their own guardian spirit song. The journeys might last from two to five nights, or until the soul of the patient is recovered.[111]

The shamans of Guatemala use a mixture of traditional Indian beliefs and Christianity, despite the fervent attempts of the Spanish to purge paganism from the Americas. The shamans call on and intervene with saints and spirits for the purposes of divination and healing, using magic stones—usually bits of ancient Mayan sculpture—as their vehicle for communication. The services of shamans, as well as "witches" who practice the blacker side of magic, are expensive for these poor people, ranging from the equivalent of fifty to a hundred dollars. The ceremonial fee covers the cost of necessary preparations and ingredients: the incense, candles, flowers, a dinner, and an immense quantity of distilled spirits, which the shaman drinks until he becomes exceedingly loquacious.[112]

The Canadian Eskimo shaman goes into a trance, journeys to the netherworld at the bottom of the sea, and visits the sea goddess Sedna to learn the causes of illness or to petition for other needs of living. Sedna is believed to control the source of food as well as all the calamities the Eskimo is likely to experience. At other times, magnificently carved and colored masks of the power animals are worn to aid in the shaman's imagery and in the contact with the animal spirits.[113]

The Crow Indians, like the Guatemalans, use rocks as medicine. These rocks, which are found and intuitively recognized as having healing qualities, are a tool for evoking visualizations. One-Child-Woman, the neglected wife of a rascal named Sees the Living Bull, found the most famous medicine rock of all. In the depths of depression, she left her camp to retreat into the mountains, and hopefully, to die. The story goes that she got a new lease on life when she found a multi-faced rock; on one side she saw her husband, on another side was the outline of a buffalo, then an eagle, and on the fourth side was a horse. She also observed that it had the marks of horse and buffalo tracks. This same rock was later noteworthy for many feats: it brought success in gambling ventures, it led war parties, proved a source of longevity for its owners, and through its visionary enhancement, provided foreknowledge of the coming cattle and European style houses.[114]

Navaho medicine has provided one of the best, and near-last, frontiers for the study of American shamanism. The sand painting is the central element in Navaho healing, and represents the spiritual and physical landscape in which a patient and illness exist, the etiology of the disease, and the mythology chosen for cure. Gladys Reichard describes the ritual as a combination of many elements, such as the medicine bundle with its sacred contents, prayer sticks made of wood and feathers, stones, tobacco, water from holy places, string, and intricate sandpaintings.[115] There is emphasis on song, prayer, body painting, sweating and emetic (the purification), and vigil for concentration and clarity of thought. During the healing ritual, the sick person sits next to the chanter and in the center of the Navaho people who have drawn together for the ceremony. Power radiates from the center to all in attendance. Throughout the long ritual, the patient is involved in symbolic drama, especially as he is encouraged to continuously develop and sustain images of the personal healing process. The songs and chants and paintings are by no means passively attended. Their mythological content must be intently concentrated upon for the power of the healing ritual to be actualized.

According to Reichard, the Navaho system combines divination with visualization. Divination is a corollary to Western medicines' diagnostic procedures. The information might come from nature, or from spirits. The Navaho determine illness by gazing at the sun, moon, or stars, by listening, or trembling. Trembling, or motion-in-the-hand, is induced during the appropriate ritual. The tremblings eventually lead to great body shudders, and the diviner enters into another state of consciousness. These are power states, and in them, the symbols for healing are visualized by the trembler. Reichard describes gazing, which may also accompany trembling, as seeing the symbol as an after-image of the heavenly body upon which concentration is focused.

While herbalists are employed by the Navaho for purely symptomatic relief, the truly curative work is accomplished by the singers or ceremonalists. The absence of the use of organic substances by these healers is regarded as a status position. Bergman, a physician who studied in a Navaho school for "medicine men," noted the memory and stamina required to perform fifty to a hundred hours of ritual chanting.

Bergman conducted an hypnosis demonstration for these healers with whom he was studying. He said that instead of looking half
asleep as they usually did during their meetings, they watched in
wide-eyed wonder (although he noted that they scarcely seemed
to be breathing). Thomas Largewhiskers, a venerated 100-year-old
medicine man, said he was surprised to see that white man knew
anything so worthwhile! The healers noted the similarity between
the hypnotic state and trembling for diagnosis, and asked Bergman
to suggest to his subject that they do some diagnostic work. Bergman
felt that was too serious a matter to play with, but agreed to ask his
Indian subject to predict the weather for the next six months. Light
rain, she predicted, followed by a dry spell of several months, and
then a good wet late summer. "I make no claim other than the truthful
reporting of facts," said Bergman. "She was precisely correct." [116]

Conclusion

What conclusions can be drawn from looking at these differing cultural manifestations? In assessing this highly subjective material,
one might best conclude that the pathway through the skylights of
consciousness is the same regardless of how and where the shamanic
voyage is begun in ordinary reality. The descriptions of the various
shamanic methods of diagnosis and healing are quite similar: entering the patient, becoming the patient, and reestablishing the sense
of connectedness with the universe. And in all traditions, all of this
is done in a state of consciousness quite different from the one used
to drive a car or to write a prescription. The cultural addenda to the
basic principles of healing are largely occasioned by whatever local
resources are present to serve as "medicine." Medicine can be defined here in two ways: first, as the vehicle of transport for the
shaman (and often the patient) to enter the requisite state of consciousness; and second, as the material symbols of the healing
state—the medicine bundles, sacred art, intrusive objects removed
from the patient, the power animal, the curing stones, and so forth.
However, as was mentioned earlier, an accomplished shaman would
theoretically require neither of these types of medicine, using instead only well-developed powers of the imagination. The symbols
and rituals that hold power culturally appear to be necessary to
open the healing mechanism for the patient, who is not as well-
schooled spiritually as the shaman.

Finally, for shamans of all genres, the distinction between body,
mind, and spirit is nil. Body is mind, and mind is spirit. Although

the terminology I have used might seem to indicate that the shamans are dealing with body, mind, and spirit as separate entities, in the literal sense, they do not. Nor do the shamans technically move from physical places to spirit realms, because they are already one and the same. Self is stone, and the stone is the universe. The shaman does not think, "Here spirit enters into matter," but "assumes spirit is always in matter, is matter—not only during the disease but from the moment of embodiment and the onset of creation itself." [117] Yet, at the same time it is not incorrect to recognize the individual qualities of body, mind, and spirit. In this system they are considered both part of each other and separate from each other, much as a tree is part of, and separate from, the earth and the sky.

To understand this total unity, it is important to realize how we are hamstrung by the limitations of English expression. The activity of consciousness and imagination is more poetry than prose, and is only imperfectly understood when language is used in its description. In describing unseen properties, the physicists resort to mathematics and visual analogies; likewise, the shamans resort to symbols and rituals. In a book such as this, however, we are bound by the limits of a language system evolved from a very specific view of reality, so the verbal expressions used here should be regarded as mere attempts to point to the nonverbal dynamics of the imagination.

2 The Golden Thread: Imagery and the History of Medicine

A golden thread has run throughout the history of the world, consecutive and continuous, the work of the best men in successive ages. From point to point it still runs, and when near you feel it as the clear and bright and searchingly irresistible light which Truth throws forth when the great minds conceive it.

Walter Moxon, Pilocereus Senilis and Other Papers, *1887.*

It might seem as though the shamanistic model of using the imagination to heal has no relevance to our modern world view. In this chapter, I will examine the history of Western medicine itself, tracing the thread of imagery in healing through the ages. To begin with, the Hippocratic Oath, the ethical code of honor still taken by every practicing physician today, is a dedication to the mythical founding family of medicine, whose contribution was a method for healing with imagination. It begins: "I swear by Apollo the Physician, by Asclepius, by Hygeia and Panacea and by all the Gods and Goddesses, making them my witnesses, that I will fulfill according to my ability and judgment this oath and this covenant."

Even though dreams and vision are universally the most common method of inquiry into the cause and cure of disease,[1] never has the inquiry been systematized and integrated into the standard cultural practice of medicine as well as during the Grecian era, when medicine's light burned as brightly as an exploding star, before its cold and dark descent through the Middle Ages.

Asclepius, the demigod honored as the figurehead of the finest

Grecian era, was represented in Homer's Iliad as an aristocrat, a physician, and a warrior king who made great contributions of ships as well as men to the Trojan War. Legend, which significantly embellished his adventures, has it that he was born of a romantic encounter between the god Apollo and a mortal woman named Coronis. Coronis double-crossed Apollo by marrying Ischys, instead, while still pregnant with Apollo's child. Apollo had the lovers put to death. As Coronis was burning on the funeral pyre, Apollo snatched his son, Asclepius, and sent him to the retreat of Chiron. Now, Chiron was a centaur charged with rearing the bastard children of the gods, and he had full knowledge of the healing arts. Asclepius was an apt pupil, and eventually his skill at saving lives was so great that Zeus became fearful the afterworld would soon be depopulated. Zeus then struck Asclepius down with a lightning bolt, and brought him into the heavens as a deity.

Asclepius had a famous healing family: his wife, Epione, soothed pain; his daughters, Hygeia and Panacea, were deities for health and treatment; and his son, Telesphoros, came to represent convalescence or rehabilitation. Asclepius himself became the patron, the demigod, and the chief representative of healing for centuries. The legend of Asclepius was merged with that of the Egyptian god of healing, Imhotep, and with the god Serapis of the Ptolemies. Historians say, "Apparently the legend was so persuasive, and Asclepius so satisfied the need for a personal, compassionate divinity, that he inherited, replaced, or merged with the power and influence of each local healing god, wherever the Asclepian rites were introduced."[2] The legend was even incorporated by Christianity, with Saints Damian and Cosmas carrying on the healing traditions.

Asclepian Dream Therapy or Divine Sleep

In separating fact from fancy, it is apparent that Asclepius was indeed an influential mortal. Over 200 temples were eventually erected throughout the area of Greece, Italy and Turkey to honor him and the practices of medicine which he fostered. These *Asclepia*, as the temples were called, were the first holistic treatment centers. They were located geographically in lovely areas, and contained baths, spas, theaters, and places for recreation and worship. All who came for treatment were accepted, regardless of their ability to pay. This policy agreed with Asclepius' basic teaching that a physician was, in the first instance, one to whom anyone in suffering or trouble could turn. The most famous of these temples are currently being excavated and reconstructed on the island of Cos (the birthplace of Hippocrates) and in Epidaurus.

Within the Asclepia, dream therapy or divine sleep, later to be called incubation sleep by Christian practitioners, reached perfection as a healing tool. Dream therapy is a prime example of the imagination as diagnostitian and healer. Most of the patients to receive this therapy were severely ill, and all the usual medicines had proven ineffective. At night, the patients went to the temple or outlying buildings to await the gods. In preparation, "the priests take the inquirer and keep him fasting from food for one day and from wine for three days to give him perfect spiritual lucidity to absorb the divine communication."[3]

The diagnosis and healing took place during that special state of consciousness immediately prior to sleep, when images come forth automatically like frames of thought projected on a movie screen. (We now call this "hypnogogic sleep.") During this sensitive, susceptible time, Asclepius purportedly would then appear as a handsome, gentle and strong healer, who either cured or advised treatment. He held a rustic staff with a serpent entwined about it—resembling the symbol of the medical profession known as the *caduceus*. (The caduceus actually has been identified much earlier even than the ancient Greeks, and the snake emblem itself is richly endowed by cross-cultural myths with significance as a healing partner.) During the dreamlike experiences in the Asclepian temples, the snakes were reported to slither over to the patient and lick on their wounds and their eyelids—an event that in most of us would at least activate the adrenal glands!

Since the temples were established well after Asclepius' lifetime, the rituals were performed by physician/priests, dressed as Asclepius, accompanied by a retinue representing his family, and even by animals such as geese, which, in addition to the serpent, were believed to have some healing ability. Moving from patient to patient, the group carried the accoutrements of the physician, such as medicines and surgical tools, and performed, or perhaps just playacted, both the standard medical treatments as well as magical rites. In the semidarkness, in the presence of the earthly representatives of healing deities, with music playing in the background, and surrounded by all the pomp and circumstance of the magnificent shrines, whatever innate healing ability the patients possessed in the face of their grave illnesses was greatly enhanced. It was a perfect situation for the imagination to go to work; and go to work it apparently did.

A story is told of a blind woman who, after being placed in a "divine sleep," visualized Asclepius admonishing her for her weak faith. Still in the dreamlike state, she became aware of Epidaurus dropping lotion into her eyes. Upon awakening, she had recovered her sight. There is some evidence that even major surgery was performed under these conditions. Many, many other cures have been ascribed to the Asclepian techniques: the blind, lame, deaf, impotent, and barren, those with varicose veins, headaches, boils, and diseases of every conceivable organ have left stone images, or votives, or written descriptions of their cures to adorn the ancient temple walls.

Aristotle, Hippocrates, Galen

Aristotle, Hippocrates, and even Galen were trained in the Asclepian tradition, and all of them were able to articulate the role that the imagination played in health. Aristotle believed that the emotional system did not function in the absence of images. Images were formed by the sensations taken in and worked upon by the *sensus communis*, or the "collective sense." These images caused changes in bodily functions, and affected both the cure and production of disease. Aristotle also suggested that the special images of the dream state were vital. He wrote in the *Parva Naturalia*, "Even scientific physicians tell us that one should pay diligent attention to dreams, and to hold this view is reasonable also for those who are not practitioners but speculative philosophers."

Hippocrates, the "Father of Medicine," symbolized the change in the practice of medicine from mystical to naturalistic principles. He believed that the physician's role was essentially to understand and assist nature, to know what humans were in relation to food, drink, occupation, and what effect each of these had upon the others. He, too, espoused the Asclepian mode of gentleness and concern, love and dignity.

Galen, whose dictums influenced the practice of medicine for no fewer than forty-five generations, was the last important pillar in the millennium of Greek medical preeminence. In fact, medicine had already begun its decline from glory some years prior to Galen, so that what was captured and practiced by medieval Europe was by no means the crowning achievement of the Greek physicians, but rather something less. Galen's influential approach was based on the Hippocratic theories of the four humors, on the concept of critical days for health (a forerunner to biorhythms), and on erroneous theories of pulse and urine function.

Galen was the first, however, to record a full-fledged description of the effect of the imagination on health, indicating that he understood the relationship between body and mind in quite a modern sense. In the absence of laboratory tests, the patient's imagery or dream content was believed to offer clinically important diagnostic information. For example, images of loss or grief related to an excess of melancholy (black bile), and images of terror or fright reflected a predominance of choler. Galen emphasized the circularity inherent in excessive humors, which then nourished corresponding images, which in turn produced an elaboration of the humor. He acknowledged the implications of the vicious cycle for therapy, and stressed the importance of breaking the cycle at some point to regain health.[4]

According to Osler, "The Greek view of man was the very antithesis of that which St. Paul enforced from the Christian world. One idea pervades thought from Homer to Lucian like an aroma—pride in the body as a whole. In the strong conviction that 'our soul in its rose mesh' is quite as much helped by flesh as flesh by soul the Greek sang his song—'For pleasant is this flesh.'" Prodicus made a statement in the fifth century, B.C.: "That which benefits human life is God." This implies a principle of unity that lends to the Greek healing arts a metaphysical flavor and goodness that in and of itself was not at odds with the Christ consciousness that was about to sweep through the Western world.

The characteristic Greek attention to physical needs and to health was put on the back burner of human priority, particularly in the West, for several hundred years. Nevertheless, Asclepius as a respected healing figure survived the Christian purge of the pagan gods—the similarities between him and Jesus were just too obvious to be overlooked. The Asclepian tradition bridged the time until the Church resurrected certain aspects of Grecian thought—including Galen's work—and made them holy. Statues of the Asclepian family, the caduceus symbol, and the Hippocratic Oath have all persisted down through the ages as a reminder that a theme of wisdom has indeed run through the history of healing—one that specifies that the healing mission must be one of love and respect for humanity. As Hippocrates stated, "Where there is love for mankind, there is love for the art of healing."

Anglo-Saxon Medicine of the Middle Ages

During the Dark or Middle Ages, there was no serious study or practice of medicine outside of the religious or folk tradition in most of the Western world. For this reason, it is exceedingly difficult to accurately chronicle the role of the imagination in medicine during the period after the Greek era until the Renaissance, even though the imagination could likely be held responsible for many cures which were accomplished. Part of the obscurity at this time comes from the fact that practitioners of both folk and religious healing regarded healing rites as mysteries to be shared only with chosen initiates and preserved only through an oral account. While the religious methods sanctioned by the Catholic church can be surmised by extrapolating from modern to vintage practice, the techniques of the folk medicine practiced by the Anglo-Saxon women have long since been legislated underground or out of existence altogether. The healing practices of the women of those years must largely be deduced from the documents obtained from the witch trials.

From piecing together facts from the historical accounts of Europe and the British Isles, it appears that the period extending from A.D. 500 through approximately 1300 could be described as most colorful and creative in the use of the imagination. The methods used go back to the dawn of civilization, and mingle with the shamanic roots of other continents. The deities invoked in the healing rituals have their counterparts in both Greek and Roman myth.

Anglo-Saxon healing was the province of wise women as well as of the Catholic church during its centuries of preeminence. Quackery, too, was declared rampant, although one would be hard pressed then, as now, to adequately discriminate "quack" from "nonquack." In any case, what little we know of the practices of these groups provides historical support and documentation for the primacy of the imagination in medical intervention, and the ability of the human body to heal itself, often in spite of the travesties visited upon it in the name of medicine.

Woman as Healer

During this era, it was the wise women who used the nonrational, intuitive aspects of the mind in a healing capacity. They provided the medicine for the masses of humanity, yet their healing arts were

banished to the fringe, first by the Church and then by the govern-
ments of Europe, England and America. The women and their fine
skills were the losers in a social and political battle for jurisdiction
over the care of the human frame. Strangely, there is no indication
from reports of their contemporaries that they were anything but
powerful and effective.

Paracelsus, the Renaissance giant of a physician and founder of
modern chemistry, credited his understanding of the laws and practices of health to his conversations with the wise women. As he
breathed life into the art of healing by defying the outmoded, deca-
dent mandate of the Grecian age in medicine, he threw his medical
books into the fire and turned to the wisdom of the women's medicine. Matilda Gage, a meticulous and inspired nineteenth-century
scribe of church and state policy relating to women, said of Paracelsus, "I make no doubt that his admirable and masterly work on
the Diseases of Women, the first written on this theme, so large,
so deep, so tender, came forth from his special experience of those
women to whom others went for help, the witches, who acted as
midwives, for never in those days was a male physician admitted to
women."[5]

Regardless of Paracelsus' and others respect for the wise women,
the witches (as they were often called) met with a notoriously bad
fate. According to some scholars, the word *witch* itself signified
superior learning or wisdom. Henry More, a learned Cambridge
graduate of the 1600's, further stated that the terminology indicated
a woman had uncommon *but not unlawful* skill. The derivation of the
English word is debated, but *wekken*, "to prophesy," or *witan*, "to
know," are candidates. The Slavonian word for witch is *vjedma*, derived from the verb "to know." A Russian term for witch is *zaharku*,
also derived from the verb *znat*, or "to know." In accordance with
the overwhelming evidence that the witch was associated with knowledge and with the practice of the ancient arts of healing, and not
with Satanic worship or evil doing, I will use the word *witch* re-
spectfully, and interchangeably with *wise woman*.

The wise women, steeped in the pagan ways, were wholly
shamanic in their regard for the unity and life of all things, and in
their attempt to use the forces of nature for healing purposes. They
knew the herbal remedies and the magic incantations, and their
ability to soothe pain and heal, commendably, survived through the
Middle Ages. Their use of natural anesthetics was valuable at a time
when most of humanity was cursed with aches of one kind or an-

other. The Solanaceous herbs, especially belladonna, eased the pains and perils of motherhood. "In childbirth, a motherly hand instilled the gentle poison, casting the mother herself into a sleep and soothing the infant's passage, after the manner of modern chloroform, into the world."[6]

The active properties of some of their strange remedies have been identified. Bufotenine, a powerful hallucinogen, has been derived from toads, an ever-popular witches' remedy. The widely used and mysterious mandrake roots contain scopolamine, and when combined with morphine can produce surgical anesthesia. Even garlic has been shown to have positive effects on the cardiovascular system. The women were clearly using empirically based treatments, treatments that had been shown to work time and time again. Their scientific acumen was described by Gage thusly: "The superior learning of witches was recognized in the widely extended belief of their ability to work miracles. The witch was in reality the profoundest thinker, the most advanced scientist of those ages."[7]

However, in surveying the wise women's storehouse of medicines, we must conclude that although a superb herbal lore existed, much cure must have relied upon the effect of the rituals and incantations upon the imagination, and not the ingredients of the potions. Excretia from various sources and the sundry parts of hanged men were used by wise women, and later by the physicians who obviously hoped to emulate their success, with a wide variety of ailments. A touch of the dead man's hand was used to cure wens; his freshly drawn blood was a specific for epilepsy. Moss growing on the skull of someone who had died so unnatural a death was a prized panacea, properly referred to as *usnea*. Cutting the tongue out of a fox, tying it up in a red cloth, and wearing it around one's neck was a remedy for cataracts. Dragon's blood, whatever substance that may have been, was used in a number of tonics.

During the years of the great plagues, which thinned the population of Europe and England to mere shadows, the special knowledge of the witches was sought even by the upper classes, albeit secretly. None of the theory-laden classes taught in the universities had prepared the physicians to cope with the epidemics, and it was widely believed that only the practitioners of the supernatural could stem the deadly tide. Practically everyone, it seemed, *believed* in the magic of the wise women, but *practicing* it had become quite risky. Anything that smacked of the supernatural was declared by the Church to be rank heresy, and punishable by the most severe means.

The wary healer needed to keep up with the contemporary rules. Paradoxically, astrology and alchemy were regarded as natural medicine; they were practiced by the physicians of the time, and were within the teachings of the Church. But the herbs and blessings administered by the midwives were considered to be the work of the devil. Woman was expected to undergo continual penance for the trespasses of Eve, and the pains of childbirth were regarded as her just desserts. Any attempt at mitigating the discomfort was viewed as a dangerous act against the Church. In any event, heresy was likely to be vicariously defined by who was practicing what on whom.

Wise Woman as Shaman

Anthropologists with cross-cultural information on shamanistic health practices have concluded the wise women (witches) were acting within the long-standing pagan tradition of European tribes whose practices were essentially shamanic. (A qualification should be made here: Not all of the women accused of practicing witchcraft were likely to have been thusly involved. The early victims may well have been sought out for their pagan beliefs, but when the witch hunt reached the height of madness, accusations ran rampant, and even the suspected women accused scores of the innocent in order to bring a swift end to their personal tortures.)

Margaret Murray, in her classic but controversial text, *The Witch Cult in Western Europe*, was the first to turn a sensitive, scientific eye to the material. She proposed that witchcraft could be traced to pre-Christian times, to a religion centered upon an ancient deity that incarnated in the form of either a man or an animal, but most often a woman. Diana, the feminine form of the Roman god Janus, was the figure upon which most of the European cults were based. Murray claimed the cults largely engaged in activities that would ensure the fertility of their crops and animals.[8] Mircea Eliade, one of the most prolific, respected scholars of the history of traditional religions, was convinced after studying Indian and Tibetan documents that the witchcraft sect could neither be the falsified creation of religion or politics, nor a demonic sect devoted to Satan. ". . . All the features associated with European witches are—with the exception of Satan and the Sabbat—claimed also by Indo-Tibetan yogis and magicians. They too are supposed to fly through the air, render themselves invisible, kill at a distance, master demons and ghosts. . . ."[9]

Eliade also points to the cults of the *benandanti* in Italy, and to

Romanian folk religion. These, too, were said to be composed of special people who fought spiritual battles in trance, flew to their assemblies, changed shape, and healed with magic. Both groups acknowledge Diana as a deity; but unlike the witches, both cults have survived without undue persecution.

Michael Harner, the anthropologist and shaman, also believes the witches were part of the shamanic tradition.[10] He points out their journeying to the upper world of the imagination, riding their broomsticks up and out of the chimney with the smoke. Harner furthermore suggests that European fairy tales were once shamanic adventure stories: Mother Goose who rode on a goose and Santa Claus who used a sleigh drawn by reindeer all fit the mode. Since the deer is universally regarded as a spirit guide into the unconscious, having eight such totems would surely make a shaman powerful.

Shamans and witches alike have a profound respect for nature, and believe in and use the interconnectedness of all things as integral to healing ritual. The idea of flying in another state of consciousness to realms where the imagination breathes freely, where work can be done to heal the social structure of the community, as well as bodies and souls, are common to both practices. But, as always when old religions are replaced, the ancient deities become devils in the new order. Even the "Horned One," the consort of the witches, has been assigned the evil role of Satan in modern religions. Instead, he probably represented the deer spirit, and wore horns as part of the holy regalia typical of the shamans in virtually every culture. (It is interesting, what we do with our symbolism. The Christ figure was often portrayed in the garb of a deer in the art of medieval England.)

Another point of comparison between the witches and the shamans is their use of drugs. The witches likely did not perform their healing rituals in drug-induced trances, which differentiates them from many of the shamans on the American continents. The drugs that they were known to use were extremely strong and dangerous. Records from the Inquisition indicated the women appeared to be comatose for days after rubbing themselves with their "flying oyl"—a combination of either henbane, datura, belladonna, or mandrake root. Death from overdose must have been quite common. Harner, in his review of this area, believes the trances were of a sort to make ritual work impossible, and the aftermath of long, deep sleep followed by amnesia were likewise incompatible with healing. Harner suggests the witches, like the Jívaro with whom he studied, used the Solanaceous hallucinogens simply to encounter the supernatural, but not to engage in any activities, such as healing rituals, which would require awareness of ordinary reality.[11]

The few reports of the administration of the flying ointment, or a reasonable facsimile, under conditions of self-experimentation indicate the drugs do induce feelings of flight as well as vivid imagery. Mixing a seventeenth century formula of belladonna, henbane and datura, Professor Will-Erich Peukert and his colleagues, after rubbing it on their foreheads, "fell into a twenty-four hour sleep in which they dreamed of wild rides, frenzied dancing, and other weird adventures of the type connected with medieval orgies."[12]

Quackery

During the Middle Ages and throughout the Renaissance, there was much concern given to quackery and the inappropriate practice of medicine. The quacks were regarded as a group separate from the physicians, and were no less condemned than the wise women. After looking over the standard cures used by all of these practitioners—dragon's blood, usnea, incantations and beseechings of a ritual order—it would seem that ferreting out who the quacks actually were might be a problem. Quackery did not (and still doesn't) relate to the techniques used, since there is a vast overlap in healing practices. Quack and physician alike may use the same procedures at once, or borrow each other's discarded repertoire.

Eric Maple in his writings on the medical history of this period suggests that quackery then, as now, related not to motive, education, practices, or deceit, but to social standing, with the quacks being members of the perennial social class known as "outsiders."[13] It was the laymen who styled themselves physicians and surgeons during the Middle Ages that did the name calling. They were the "insiders" by virtue of their having organized into guilds, whereby barbers and surgeons, physicians and apothecaries united together on the basis of the similarities of their tools. They were unschooled for the most part, and deeply wedded to the concepts of magic. Care must therefore be taken in determining what is real medicine and what is quackery; otherwise we fall into the trap of damning our roots and future.

Shrine and Relic Cures

In addition to the wise women, the lay physicians and surgeons, and the various quacks, the other class of health providers during the early Christian era in the West was the priesthood, which was adamant that religious faith alone should be the cure. The advent of Christianity affected the practice of medicine in such a way that some scholars blame it for bringing about the darkest days in health care. The pagans (Greeks, Romans, and Egyptians, particularly) had elevated the art of healing to a height it would not see again for centuries. As Christianity spread its own gospel, all that was pagan, including the pagan practice of medicine, had to fall by the wayside. The theory was advanced by the Church that disease was caused by Satan, not by the pagan spirits; therefore, pagan medicine could have no role in its exorcism. In other words, the Church expunged the exquisite surgical and herbal skills of the Greeks from the roster of available treatments and substituted, instead, frequently brutal practices such as mortifying the flesh. This brought the standard practice of physical medicine to an all-time low. (By the thirteenth century, some of this had changed as a result of the writings of St. Thomas Aquinas, who reformulated Aristotelian thought, making it impregnable doctrine throughout the duration of the Middle Ages. The medicine of Aristotle, Hippocrates and Galen, as much of it as could be interpreted after centuries of intellectual and medical stagnation, rode with this tide.)

On the other hand, with the decline of physical medicine, medicine of the imagination flourished. The treatments of choice specified by the early Church were medicines of the imagination in every sense: shrine cures, processions and pilgrimages to holy places, relics of saints and martyrs. These latter were sold at considerable gain for the coffers of the Church, as Martin Luther was later to point out in a fit of pique that gave Christianity a supreme test of divisiveness. Holy relics apparently had healing power, notwithstanding the fact that the majority were no doubt outright fakes. According to records, "The shrine of St. Ursula at Cologne retained its popularity even after the skeletons of the eleven thousand virgins had been proved to be those of males" and the "miraculous bones of the blessed St. Rosalia at Palermo were later discovered to be that of a goat." [14]

During the decline of the medieval period, saints increasingly took on areas of specialty, either because of their dedication to certain populations, or for more tenuous reasons. St. Teresa of Avila became protectress of cardiac patients because an angel had supposedly shot an arrow through her own heart. There were fertility, leprosy, and plague specialists. Drugs, if we might refer to them as such, were the scrapings from the gravestones of these holy men and women, water from wells near their shrines, or dirt where their feet had trod. These substances were mixed into potions or worn as amulets. Testimonials for healing proliferated.

Incubation or Divine Sleep of the Saints

The golden thread of healing with the imagination that was associated with the Asclepian temples of Turkey and Greece remained intact, despite the marked influence of the Church, the guilded physicians, and the folk healers. Instead of Asclepius and his retinue, the miracles of healing were attributed to Saints Cosmas and Damian, twins who met a grotesque martyrdom during the Diocletian persecution (278 A.D.). They later became patron saints for the entire healing profession of Western civilization. These men worked incessantly, and provided their services without fee, in hopes of gaining converts to Christianity. Churches dedicated to their names were open day and night for the care of the sick, using the method of *incubatio*, or incubation sleep, modeled after the divine sleep cures of the Greeks. During the twilight state between sleep and wakefulness, the patients would have images of the revered healers, who would provide diagnostic information and administer cures.

The credentials of the techniques were established and embellished in legend, increasing the expectancy of the patients and ripening their readiness for cure. One of the most famous stories told (and preserved in an anonymous work of art displayed at the Prado in Madrid) concerns a man with cancer of the leg who sought a miracle from the saints. He entered into a church dedicated to Cosmas and Damian and, while praying, fell into the appropriate state of near sleep. Cosmas and Damian appeared to him, as if in a dream. After diagnosing the problem, they amputated the gangrenous limb; then, looking about for a replacement, they could only find a black man entombed in the church to serve as a donor. The recipient of the holy ministrations awoke, noted his legs were of two different colors, but functioning quite well, and went about his business. Regardless of the element of exaggeration in the miracles, the reputation of the saints expanded rapidly, and their names and works gained importance for the physicians, surgeons, and the apothecaries and barbers.[15]

Incubation sleep practices were continued in the Christian churches in England until the present, and had a perpetual reputation for effecting exceptional cures. Thus, the methods of the shamans and the wise women—healing in nonordinary reality and invoking visions of spirit guides—has been a part of Christianity since its inception. Only the names have been changed.

The Official End of Folk-Medicine

A discussion of the end of the folk medicine tradition is in order here. This might seem to be a digression from the historical description of healing practices that evoked the power of the imagination, but in fact, the following events initiated the ostracism of such practices, which has characterized the medicine of Western civilization ever since the sixteenth century. In Russia, Eastern Europe, Asia, certainly in South and Central America, viable shamanic traditions continue to hold forth, often despite suppression and official denial of their existence. Such is not the case for the medical lineage of the United States, which generally includes the English and Western European traditions. (I am not ignoring the scattered instances of groups, such as Wicca, which claim to practice the ancient Celtic healing rituals. They are not integrated into the culture, nor do they reflect even a minority attitude of the culture.)

In 1518, physicians and surgeons bound themselves together in an organized structure, and the College of Physicians was established. The Acts of Incorporation clearly defined who could and could not practice medicine. The outsiders were common artificers such as "smyths, wevers, and women," who were accused of being grossly ignorant, and of using sorcery and witchcraft and noxious medications, to the high displeasure of God. Note that men were excluded from medicine on the condition of their profession, women on the basis of their sex.

Then, the economic reality of creating an elite profession hit the peasantry with full force. The licensed physicians and surgeons were not at all interested in treating charity cases. King Henry VIII intervened on behalf of the hordes of ailing poor, and decreed that the nonlicensed healers could cure all maladies on the surface of the body, but only with plasters, poultices and ointments. Thus magic, as well as surgery and medicine, was expressly forbidden to the folk healers by this document, which became known as the *Quack's Charter*.

To further compound the problems of keeping medicine exclusive, England, by virtue of her separation from Rome, had to deal with unemployed monks who flooded the job market after the monastaries closed. Doctoring was a direction many headed towards, some with a hefty resume of nursing experience, some with a knowledge of faith healing, and some in sheer desperation. One, a Mr. Thomas Pail, admitted, "I have no other means left for my maintenance but to turn physician. God he knows how many lives it will cost."[16]

The Fate of the Wise Women

In the midst of the atmosphere of change brought about by the issuance of the official mandates determining who should minister to the sick—and not coincidentally—one of the saddest events in the history of women and healing began: the great witch hunt. It was inordinately successful in eliminating womens' influence on the healing arts up to the present day. In fact, it was inordinately successful in eliminating women, period. Estimates are that anywhere from a few hundred thousand to nine million women were murdered between the years 1500 and 1650, many of them for the suspicioned practice of medicine. Nine hundred women were destroyed in one year in the quiet university town of Wurzburg, Germany, and a hundred in the vicinity of Como, Italy. At Toulouse, four hundred were killed in one day, and in the Bishopric of Trier, in 1585, two villages were left with only one woman each.

The women were accused of causing all the ills of Europe, England, and America. If the licensed physicians failed to cure, a witch was blamed. If a cow's milk dried up, a witch was blamed. Women were tortured by the most ingenious means, perfected by the Holy Inquisition and carried out with Calvinistic zeal, until they confessed to all imaginable horrors: having sexual intercourse with the devil, raising tempests, and feasting upon dead babies. The alleged crimes of the witches can be classified into three broad categories. First, were sexual crimes against men. The treatise that was widely used in the trials, *The Malleus Maleficarum* (The Witches Hammer), written in 1486 by Heinrich Kramer and James Sprenger, stated that "all witchcraft comes from carnal lust which is in women insatiable." Their second major offense was that of being organized, which may or may not have been true. They may have led peasant rebellions, and there is evidence they convened in village groups. Third, and most pertinent, they were accused of having the magical power to affect health, both in their ability to heal as well as to cause illness and death.[17]

Distinguishing between good and bad witches, or "white" and "black" magic, was not at issue. In fact, the legal distinction was dropped in 1563 in Scotland, where the good witches were seen as at least as great a threat as the bad. William Perkins, a leading witch hunter, declared that the "good witch was a more horrible and detestable monster than the bad," and, "if death be due to any . . . then a thousand deaths of right belong to the good witch."[18] It was further declared that it would be a thousand times better for the land if all the witches, but especially the blessing (good) witch, might suffer death. Kramer and Sprenger also voiced their opinion that the midwives did more harm to the Catholic church than anyone else.

According to Ehrenreich and English in their book, *Witches, Midwives, and Nurses: A History of Women Healers*, the Church saw its attack on the witch healers as an attack on magic, but not on medicine. "The greater their satanic powers to help themselves, the less they were dependent on God and the Church and the more they were potentially able to use their powers against God's order." Magic charms were not spurned as any less effective than prayer, "but prayer was Church sanctioned and controlled while incantations and charms were not." It seems that one could readily distinguish God's cures from the devil's, because God worked through the priests and doctors rather than through the women.

The fury against women became self-perpetuating. The original charges were obscured, and women were attacked wholesale for the sole crime of not having been born male. Eventually, only those of noble blood were even half safe. We have seen such an unreasoned panic twice during this century: once in Nazi Germany, and once during the McCarthy years of Communist hunting in the United States. In both instances, unlike the witches, the victims were occasionally able to survive to tell their side of the story and be vindicated.

Unsolved Riddles

Both the fate of the witches and their practices are of great interest in considering the role of the imagination in health: their fate is relevant because it has forever put a restraint on Western civilization's attitude toward both women and their medicine of the imagination; and their practices are pertinent because of their enduring repute.

Not all scholars would agree with the position that the women were practicing effective medicine, or indeed, that they were practicing medicine at all. Gregary Zilboorg, a modern authority, examined the retrospective information on the witches and concluded one should seriously consider the original nature of the charges against them; that is, that the witches were "heretical; they actually sinned against the Sacraments . . . actually either rebelled against or were afraid of the sign of the Cross—all this while mentally sick, of course."[19] This position is one that has continued to be favored by the Church, perhaps to absolve historical guilt. It is of note that Zilboorg's ideas on insanity have also been supported by modern psychiatrists. Nowhere in the modern psychiatric literature has mental illness been proposed in conjunction with the behavior of the persecutors.

Other historians, in particular Marvin Harris, believe there were no real crimes, nor any witches either; but rather that all charges against the women were concoctions on the part of nobility to devise a scapegoat for the problems facing Europe during the times of peasant rebellions, the rash of messianic movements, and the upheaval of the Reformation.[20] Mary Daly, an avowed radical feminist, proposes that the witchcraze was a sexist movement in the same category with footbinding, clitoridectomy, and the unnecessary prescription and mutilative surgery performed on women in the civilized world.[21]

Economic issues surely contributed provocation to the hunt. First, consider the economic threat to the established or guilded practitioners of medicine in a market flooded with healers. The women were significantly more vulnerable to ostracism than either the priest or physician networks. And even though the women were poorly paid for their services (if paid at all), their superior knowledge and reputation were surely a grave threat. Further, financial booty was paid to the court from the accused womens' estates to cover the cost of the trials, and the witch hunters earned large sums each time they identified a witch who was eventually accused. The torturers and executioners earned a good living also.[22] And finally, all worldly belongings of the woman became the property of the Church.

Woman as Nature

On a more philosophical note, the women healers were ensnared in the fissures created by the shifting paradigm of science. As humanity began its preparations for the new world view that would encompass the scientific method, all that was irrational and all that was intuitive was subject to being purged. Women's science and women's medicine were prime targets. Women, from the beginning of time, were believed to hold the secrets of life within their very being. And with these mysteries, they gave birth and birthed, healed and nourished the growth of living things. For these life-giving, life-saving skills, they were first deified and then tortured. Did women really have sufficient intuitive knowledge of natural law to alter the course of a storm or a life? The Church fathers thought so, as did the population at large.

What has been witnessed over the centuries is a fanciful mixing of metaphors, such that Woman as Nature and Nature as Woman became inseparable. During the great times of change leading into and extending through the Renaissance, both were to be stripped and their inner parts revealed. Nature/Woman was being forced to confess her knowledge. (In England, jurors and others in attendance at the trials gang-raped the women before the hearings. The practice was so common it was not even included as part of the documentation of torture, but rather as a simple trial preliminary event.) A case in point comes from the remarks of Sir Francis Bacon, the great empiricist whose work is credited with uniting science and technology. In describing his new methods of investigation, he stated that nature had to be "hounded in her wanderings," "bound into service," and made a "slave," and that the aim of science was to "torture nature's secrets from her."[23] Bacon seems to have been inspired by the witch trials over which he presided as attorney general for King James I. Capra states, "Indeed, his view of nature as a female whose secrets have to be tortured from her with the help of mechanical devices is strongly suggestive of the widespread torture of women in the witch trials of the early seventeenth century. Bacon's work thus represents an outstanding example of the influence of patriarchal attitudes on scientific thought."[24]

It was not purely "femaleness" that was so blatantly challenged with regard to the role of women in science and medicine. It was, rather, that the qualities traditionally associated with women posed a threat to what was eventually to become known as the Newtonian world view, i.e., the concept that the body, as well as the universe, was a great machine. Intuition, feelings, nonrational thought, holism, nurturance, and the imagination have scant place in the thought mode of a universe made of cogs and wheels. In fact, it is generally believed that science advanced from magical thinking to its current status principally because this "baggage" was cast aside. Yet, the emerging scientific understanding in the fields of physics, biochemistry and physiology suggest something quite different. It now seems that the remaining mysteries of life, and more practically, improvement in the conditions of living on this planet, will be out of reach until we enter an era that acknowledges precisely those feminine qualities as both rightful and appropriate to the pursuit of science.

The ostracism of the shamanic aspect of women's medicine, at first economic and political in nature, later became necessary because science could not account for what appeared to be transpersonal phenomena. They were therefore legislated out of existence. Modern developments in science now suggest this decision was inappropriate. In Chapter 4, I will present evidence that substantiates the effectiveness of the imagination, using information from basic science, without recourse to supernatural interpretation.

The Renaissance Period of Paracelsus

Even though it was extremely dangerous for women to practice healing, the imagination that so permeated their techniques continued to be incorporated into medicine during the Renaissance. It became associated with avant garde, but licensed, medical practice primarily through the work of Paracelsus. One of the most outrageous physicians of his or any other time, Paracelsus has been referred to by his biographers as the stormy petrel of medicine, medicine's Luther, an arch-charlatan, drunken quack, the founder of modern chemistry, and the Renaissance Christ of Healing. He cured and quarreled and made men think, as Osler said, "stirring the pool as had not been done for fifteen centuries."[25]

Paracelsus committed the barbaric and unforgiveable act of giving his lectures in German, his native tongue, instead of the usual Latin. He further demonstrated his disdain for years of tradition, albeit unmarred by progress, by building a bonfire and burning the *Canon*, the bible of medicine of his time. He spoke out boldly for independent judgment among physicians, and for learning medicine by providing actual bedside care. His contemporaries railed against him; his patients adored him—and for good reason. Opium, with its blessed anesthetic properties, was brought back from the Orient and stored in the head of his cane, to ease what must have been unspeakable discomforts of that time. Recall that these were the days when ships were sent halfway around the world on the famous "cinnamon trade routes" to obtain the spice to treat wounds—not to heal them, but to cover the stench of putrid flesh. So much for the good old days. Rather than turning a deaf ear, or worse, ridiculing the people's medicine, Paracelsus listened to the wise women and the folk healers, and incorporated their knowledge into his own medicine—particularly obstetrics, a field that male doctors practiced literally in the dark, since they were rarely afforded even a peek at the mother-to-be's anatomy during labor and delivery.

Paracelsus reiterated the theme, so reminiscent of the ancient Greeks, that three *principias* were incorporated into humanity: the spiritual, the physical, and mentalistic phenomena. Stoddart, in 1911, paraphrased Paracelsus thusly: "Man is his own doctor and finds proper healing herbs in his own garden; the physician is in ourselves, and in our own nature are all things that we need."[26]

On the subject of the imagination, Paracelsus is quoted as having said the following: "Man has a visible and an invisible workshop. The visible one is his body, the invisible one is imagination (mind). . . . The imagination is sun in the soul of man. . . . The spirit is the master, imagination the tool, and the body the plastic material. . . . The power of the imagination is a great factor in medicine. It may produce diseases . . . and it may cure them. . . . Ills of the body may be cured by physical remedies or by the power of the spirit acting through the soul."[27]

Theorizing on the Imagination: Pre-Descartes

In order to understand the theorizing of the pre-Cartesian physicians, one must remember that for them, as well as for the shamanic and wise women healers, images were as much a physiological reality as any of the other body functions. They had no direct knowledge of anatomy and physiology either, since they were forced to speculate upon them in the absence of technologically advanced methods of measurement and observation. McMahon, who has reviewed the role of the imagination during several eras in history, stated the belief system of that time: "When an image became an obsession it pervaded the body, bound up the heart, clutched at the sinews and vessels, and directed the flesh according to its own inclination. Soon its essence became manifest in its victim's complexion, countenance, posture, and gait. Imagination had greater powers of control than sensation, and thus, anticipation of a feared event was more damaging than the event itself; horror of death killed with the same authenticity as an externally inflicted wound. A strong imagination of a particular malady, such as fever, paralysis or suffocation, was sufficient to produce its symptoms."[28]

Pre-Cartesian medical thinking was invariably holistic, and the tenet of the inseparability of mind, body, and spirit in concerns of health care was consonant with the existing world view. When the world view changed to incorporate the Cartesian model of dualism— the separation of the functions of mind from the stuff of the body— the holistic approach became logically inconsistent. Descartes himself asserted that there was nothing included in the concept of the body that belonged to the mind, and likewise nothing in the mind that belonged to the body.[29] Now implicit permission was given to dissect, bisect, examine, and otherwise invade the human body without fear of damage to the soul. The trade-off was that, in the core practice of medicine, imagery had lost its status.

3 The Shaman/ Scientist: Uses of Imagery in Modern Medicine

It is a common fate of all knowledge to begin as heresy and end as orthodoxy.

Thomas Huxley

Following the Renaissance, and until very recently, the systematic use of imagery was considered absolutely tangential to the established view of medicine. Now, practices that bear vestiges of the shamans' knowledge can be observed in modern medical settings. These techniques, which rely upon the power of the imagination, are rarely credited as being essential to the practice of technological medicine, but they are at least considered useful to the patients' psychological well-being.

In order for the imagination to move from its current adjunctive role in medicine and be awarded the stature achieved in the shamanic system of healing, two factors must be in place. First, a body of solid, convincing research must be generated to support the role of the imagination in total health. The burden of proof and the responsibility for the research rests with those who support the reintegration of the imagination in health care, not with those scientists who choose to sustain the status quo of allopathic medicine. Second, those who heal in the imaginary realms must also understand and speak the language of the scientist in order to establish credibility and be embraced within the medical community. The finest medicine will be practiced by those who take the best from the shaman and from the scientist.

This chapter describes some of the techniques employed by individuals who are trying to bring the two worlds together. We could say these individuals are practicing shaman/scientists. Whenever possible, documentation of the results of clinical practice are provided, together with case material. These modern practitioners use imagery in essentially three ways: as diagnosis, as therapy, and as a mental rehearsal to relieve the pain and anxiety associated with medical conditions.

The modern shaman/scientists, unlike their predecessors in the healing arts, typically do not claim to be operating in the transpersonal mode of imaginary healing. Rather, they are likely to envision themselves as teachers or guides, with any healing or diagnostic benefit coming from within the patients themselves. They can best be generalized as ascribing to the preverbal notion of healing with the imagination, regarding it as a natural, but often latent, human ability. Transpersonal healing may well be entertained by the shaman/scientists as viable in certain clinical applications, but it does not form the theoretical basis for the tools and techniques of the imagination that are currently being integrated into medical settings.

The Image as Part of All Health Care

Before discussing specific tools and techniques of imagery practice, I would like to emphasize the tacit role imagery plays even in the most orthodox of Western medical practices. The image is an ever-present variable in all matters of health. It may not be acknowledged, or manipulated, or used in any systematic way in treatment or diagnosis, but it is there, nevertheless, as a critical determinant of health. Imagery is not only a natural concomitant to all healing, but is involved in every interaction health care professionals have with their patients.

To begin with, when bodily sensations come to awareness, particularly if they are alarming, an image of an internal landscape is created. Just like the physicians of the fifteenth century, who had no machines to scan brains, to x-ray bones or to measure blood components, we too form mental images through a kind of cognitive assessment of symptoms. Consider the following rather common scenario, where relatively harmless symptoms become signals of impending doom as a function of our vivid imagination:

"Hey, there's a tickle in my throat I hadn't noticed before. I wonder what that means? Maybe I'm getting a cold. Last time I got a cold, that's what I remember feeling before my throat got really sore. Let me see what's going on there again." At this point, we usually focus intently upon the sensation, noting where the problem is located, how widespread the feeling is, and appraising the situation. "Well, it doesn't really hurt, but it must mean something." Then, a flood of alternative diagnoses pours through our minds. "It could be that I sat in that smoky room too long last night. Or maybe I burned myself on that hot coffee. Could just be the weather. Allergies. Nah, it's probably nothing. (Pause.) It might be cancer. What if it's cancer?" Usually there is an avalanche of images here, which we try to put quickly out of our minds. "Maybe I'll just wait a day or so and go have it looked at." In the meantime, until it gets worse, it goes away (which most things eventually do), or until we forget about it, some sort of mental activity continues, with thought pictures being formulated until one is settled upon which is in accordance with our private diagnosis.

Supposing the tickle turns into a burn. Your throat feels tight, it hurts to swallow, and you're running a fever. It is nothing really unusual, but after three days you're not much better. You trundle off to the doctor, who peers wisely into your mouth with his trusty penlight. "Hmm," he says; "hmm," again. You wonder, in your vastly weakened and vulnerable state, "Why doesn't he say something? I know. He's never seen diphtheria in an adult." Finally, he gives his best guess. "It looks like you've got a pair of abcessed tonsils." "Oh, gag," you think. "I didn't even know I still had tonsils—and abcessed, yet." Now the visual component kicks in. The last abcess you saw was a boil on the neck of the guy sitting in front of you in ninth grade Civics class. You recall how, those many years ago, you watched with fascinated revulsion as it reddened, grew, finally erupted, and left a crater that took the rest of the semester to heal. You clutch at your throat, wondering just which disgusting stage of abcess your tonsils have reached.

The image takes possession of you. Your throat gets noticeably tighter, your mouth fills with saliva. Your heart flutters in your chest. Maybe you'll never be able to swallow again. Maybe the darn thing will get so big you'll just choke to death. You do your best not to think of it popping and draining. Nausea sweeps over you as you grab the sides of the examining table. The doctor continues, "Nothing serious, we should have it cleared up in a day or so," as he reaches for his prescription pad. You smile wanly, swallow, and notice with some embarrassment that you've just genuflected slightly. Within a few seconds, you have returned from having one foot in the grave to near recovery.

Had the physician's immediate comments been of a more serious nature, the situation above would have had all the potential components of voodoo death. Images are so readily translated into physical change that dying from having been given a feared diagnosis by a credible physician is just as feasible as a hex death is to a cursed Haitian. Such cases are no longer questioned by the medical community, and many have been reported in the scientific literature.

One of my husband's early experiences with the murderous power of the imagination came when he witnessed a woman who had just had a breast biopsy given the diagnosis of breast cancer in its early stages. She died within hours, as the family and amazed staff stood around her bed. What was the cause of death? Certainly not cancer. Cancer in its early stages doesn't kill. More than likely it was something that would never appear on a coroner's report: death from the workings of the imagination. This woman had nursed her mother through a long and painful death from the same disease, and had vehemently maintained that she would never let herself get into a similar situation. As she mentally processed the diagnosis, her body obviously shut down its vital functions.

On the other hand, virtually everyone who has had contact with the medical world has at least one story of a patient who, after the surgeon examined the ailing organ, was "closed up" and sent home to die. For one reason or another, people occasionally don't understand that their diagnosis is supposed to be fatal. Either they refuse to listen, or they simply mishear what is being told them, or else their "belief" in the curative powers of surgery itself is so strong that they are incapable of understanding anything else. Such people survive against all odds; they go back to the business of living, and may not be discovered until years later when they come back into the medical system with other problems.

One such example was a woman brought to the county hospital in Dallas. She was comatose on admission, paralyzed, and diagnosed with a massive brain tumor. Her thirteen-year-old son had been trying to care for her for several weeks in their small mobile home before someone discovered their plight and called an ambulance. The surgeon "debulked" the tumor (removed as much as safely possible), and since she was regarded as very close to death, neither radiation nor chemotherapy were attempted. She did receive some physical therapy to help make her more comfortable.

Instead of dying, the sick woman got stronger and more alert daily. When it began to look as if she might go home, biofeedback was prescribed to help retrain the function in her leg. As her biofeedback therapist, I was able to observe her progress over the course of one-and-a-half years. At the end of that period, she had no evidence of tumor. What was left after surgery had been nicely cleaned up and removed by her own immune system. She was walking with a cane and a short leg brace when she made her visits to the clinic, but at home where she was more sure of her footing she used neither.

This was an intelligent woman with a great deal of worldly sense, but only moderately educated. The word "tumor" didn't necessarily imply a deadly cancer or malignancy, nor anything that couldn't be overcome with the same determination she'd used all her life to make her way in the world. She was well into her fifties and had been the sole support of a teenage son and an invalid mother. Trials and tribulations were no strangers. Her images were of recovery, not death, and she defied the odds. When I saw her last she was extremely involved in her organic garden and had even been out dancing a few times.

In the introduction to Norman Cousins' book *The Healing Heart*, Bernard Lown wrote of his experience as a physician specializing in cardiology, and addressed the power words have not only to smite but to heal, as well. He provided an example of a critically ill patient whose cardiac muscle was irreparably compromised and for whom all therapeutic means had been exhausted. During rounds, Lown mentioned to the staff that the patient had a "wholesome gallop," actually a sign of significant pathology, and usually indicative of a failing heart. Several months later the patient came for a check up in a remarkable state of recovery. He told Dr. Lown that he knew what got him better and exactly when it occurred. ". . . Thursday morning, when you entered with your troops, something happened that changed everything. You listened to my heart; you seemed pleased by the findings and announced to all those standing about my bed that I had a 'wholesome gallop.'" The gentleman then went on to reason that he must have a lot of kick to his heart and therefore could not be dying. He knew instantly that he would recover.[1] The words, conveying to the patient an image of a horse that still had "kick" to it, were obviously responsible for his new state of health.

Further evidence for the role of the imagination in disease comes from studies showing that those who cannot comprehend the messages conveyed by society and its medicine die of different causes that those who can. In a recent study, Ira Collerain, Pat Craig, and I went to the computerized records listing the cause of death among the mentally retarded and emotionally disturbed individuals in the state of Texas for a four-year period. The death rates from cancer in this group are consistently significantly low: Only about 4% of deaths are from cancer, whereas in the population at large, the incidence ranges from 15–18%.[2] Studies have reported similar results in the United States as well as in the United Kingdom and in Greece. A most recent study in Romania confirmed the findings, with 7% of the deaths in a mental institution being attributed to cancer as compared with 13% in the whole population.[3] (These differences could have happened by chance only once in 1,000 times, according to the statistics.) Furthermore, not one case of leukemia was recorded between the years 1925–1978.

The clinical observations coming from the institutions where these individuals live suggest they often do grow lumps of one kind or another, but by the time the lumps are biopsied, they're found to be benign. After my study was published, a physician whose speciality was radiation oncology wrote to me, confirming the results with his clinical experience. He'd taken a position in a new cancer treatment center on the East Coast, which was designed to serve several of the state residential facilities for the mentally handicapped. He said that much to his and everyone else's surprise, the center was significantly underutilized—there just wasn't any cancer to treat.

A rash of studies has been published since 1976 showing the immune system of schizophrenics to be different in many respects than that of nonschizophrenics.[4] Certain aspects of their immunology appear to be more competent than normal, others less. The notion of a biochemical basis for protection against cancer and other immune and autoimmune disorders does not negate the possibility that cognitive factors also enter into the picture, nor does it explain the similar findings with mental retardation and other types of mental disorders.

Is the natural course of disease different when there's an absence of fear and no images of death? These studies would point to such a conclusion. The ethical questions are then posed: If people are dying from the diagnosis of the disease and not the disease itself, should they be kept in the dark regarding the condition of their health? Should information be locked up so only the high sheriffs of medicine have access to it? Can part of the blame for the epidemics of civilization be placed upon the mass media and educators like myself who keep trying to popularize the idea that people should be responsible for their own health? Emphatically, no. Diagnoses are whimsical names, culturally determined, and have very little absolute meaning or power in and of themselves. It is not the diagnosis that kills (or cures), but the expectations and images accompanying it. It's not *what* the patients are told that is so critical to health, it is *how* they're told, how they are assisted in dealing with the diagnosis, and obviously how they choose to receive the message within the context of their own belief system.

My own patients have brought the point home to me time and again: The medical profession is omnipotent in creating imagery. The images can determine life or death independently of any medical intervention. Needless to say, the responsibility should not be taken lightly, but I'm afraid it often is.

One of my most enlightened patients was a thirty-eight-year-old woman, diagnosed with cancer of the breast. She was told by her first surgeon that, in effect, she should "make her peace" and live what life was left to her as well as she could. Even though cancer had also been found in many lymph nodes, the prognosis for five-year survival and even cure is rather optimistic compared to other types of cancer. His was an unnecessarily grim pronouncement.

This woman, trained as a nurse and family therapist, knew she didn't have to, indeed could not, live with such an attitude. She chose to exercise her option: She looked for another physician, one who held out life to her instead of death. She found one who supported her need for hope, as well as her massive search for all possible alternative remedies. He said things to her like, "You and I will fight this thing together." "You're young and healthy and stand a good chance to live forty more years at least." Such simple statements, yet they have the power to chase away the horrible impending sense of doom that usually strikes in the middle of the night.

The physician she chose didn't practice alternative types of therapy. Neither did he quite understand the imagery techniques she was so dedicated to, but he did recognize they were of significant importance to her and was supportive nevertheless. She told him that she personally had called Dr. Linus Pauling in California and his colleagues in Scotland, and that she was following their recommendations for Vitamin C therapy. For this, he gave his tacit approval. He followed her through a course of highly toxic chemotherapy, which caused none of the usual side effects except hair loss. A second "prophylactic" mastectomy was recommended in view of her chronic breast disease and high risk for additional cancer. The additional surgery was quite acceptable to her and she recovered completely in three days. Doctor and patient have continued to be partners in the effort, with never the slightest innuendo from him that she might succumb despite their efforts.

Images are also created by statistics, such as those published by the American Cancer Society, the National Cancer Institute, and publicly funded researchers. Patients nearly always ask, when given a diagnosis of severe disease, "How long do I have?" First of all, that's not a fair question to ask of any mortal. But secondly, answers need to be carefully couched to reflect the truth. Usually, a range is given that is crudely derived from median life expectancy, or the point at which 50% of the patients have died and 50% are still alive, given the variables in the condition. "You have six months, maybe a year at the outside," is a common phrase. In my experience, patients tend to comply quite well with their personal sentence. The tragedy is that a range around the median is an absolutely incorrect picture. The statistics that get reported are often collected from charity patients who subject themselves to studies in order to get free medical care. Poor people with cancer simply don't live as long as the well-to-do, and the statistics are therefore skewed.[5] Furthermore, using the range around the average is only part of the description of the course of the disease.

For example, one of my patients, whom I'll call Jan, is also a medical writer with a special interest in immunology and in cancer. Not long ago she was diagnosed with a brain tumor and told she probably had six months to live. Indeed, that is the *average* or *median* life expectancy, based on tables provided by the National Cancer Institute. However, based on information from these same tables, 38% of all patients in her age group can be expected to live for three years, and beyond that, 27% live at least ten years, and are well past the point of being declared cured. When we looked at these tables together, she said incredulously, "I've got it made!" Prior to that she had become so anxious that her emotional behavior was becoming more detrimental to her well-being than the tumor itself. Out of fear of having seizures, she pleaded for high doses of Dilantin until she became toxic and confused. She carried a huge blue sedative around with her, which she nibbled on whenever she felt a seizure imminent. It was her security blanket. Although she knew full well it couldn't get into her blood stream fast enough to abort the seizure, still it worked. Her uncontrolled crying and severe depression were probably more related to the massive doses of Valium than to her situation. She also went through incredible personal changes trying to make her life "right." The stress from so many changes, the over-medication, and the anxiety were hopelessly intertwined with the effects of the tumor itself.

Following our new reading of the statistics and support from the team at the clinic where my husband and I treated her, she began thinking and acting like a healthy person again. Within two days her speech cleared, her memory improved, and a persistent cough disappeared. She insisted on a program of physical therapy to help strengthen her weak arm and hand, and requested that her high doses of tranquilizers and sleeping pills be reduced. The neurologist working in consultation with us was astounded at her rapid progress. "It's amazing what can happen when fear is controlled," the doctor said. We have no idea whether her tumor was also shrinking, since the brain scans were not so precise. The problems believed to be related to the tumor and surrounding edema were certainly diminished.

Then Jan tentatively decided to become a subject in a new medical experiment. She was heartily encouraged to do this by a well-meaning family and a physician who knew of no other treatment. It was held out to her as her only hope. She went for an evaluation, and the doctors at the medical center where the experiment was being conducted were willing to take her on. I stressed the importance of her studying the treatment well, of reading articles if she could find them, and then asking the physicians the important questions about posttreatment survival, complications, etc. I offered to help her interpret the statistics. In following through on this advice, she called another major medical center where the doctor worked who had pioneered the study, hoping to talk with him personally. Instead, an assistant (not a physician) came to the phone and assured Jan she was only buying time. Even though she had never seen Jan, and knew nothing of the specifics of her medical condition, she went on to discuss quality of life, and to explain to Jan in some detail how she would die: painlessly, with no awareness of her surroundings.

It was a criminal act, although probably well-intended, and could have had dire consequences if the assistant had been more of an authority figure to Jan. Nevertheless, after Jan hung up the telephone, she immediately decompensated. Her way of dealing with her anxieties was to call upon her support network and talk for hours. When she called me, she asked whether I had known even one person with her disease who survived. It was an old question, and she knew the answer, but she wanted to hear what I call the "healing stories" over and over again to chase away the black doubts. After hours of turmoil, she luckily happened to remember the name of a young resident who was working in the hospital where she was to receive treatment. Having the presence of mind to find his home telephone number, she was again reassured. He said "Your tumor is quite small." No one had told her that before. He also told her it was the kind of tumor known to be sensitive to the treatment they would administer—more new information. She made the final decision then and there to participate in the study.

Later, Jan sent an eloquent letter to the assistant who had given her a death sentence long distance. Jan wrote that she really did not intend to die, but in the event that death was to be imminent, it would be neither easy nor painless, as she had been told. Relinquishing the life she cherished, leaving a young daughter, and cancelling her own hopes and dreams would indeed produce the greatest imaginable psychic pain. Without her positive support network and her own determination, Jan could well have died much before now—not of the tumor, but from either fright or hopelessness.

The Placebo Effect

When the imagination is considered as the ultimate healer, aspects of what has become known as the "placebo effect" are being addressed. *Placebo effect* is just another descriptor for a physical change that happens in the absence of any known or accepted medical intervention. The placebo effect comes about because of the imagination; but it isn't synonymous with the imagination itself. Its tenacious presence in clinical studies of drugs and surgery provides ample proof for the effect of the mind on body chemistry.

The word *placebo* is derived from a Latin word meaning "I will please." Theoretically, it can be any dummy preparation or surgical procedure that has been classified as inert. The definition is becoming ludicrous, because absolutely nothing that is taken into the body accompanied by conscious thought is chemically inert. When a substance is chemically inert, it cannot react to form compounds. Every thought is accompanied by electrochemical change; that's what thinking is—electrochemical change. So if you take a pill, and you feel that it's going to cure you, the pill is metabolized in a very different environment than if you think the pill is poison. That's a crude way of summarizing the very exciting research that is now going on regarding the biochemical aspects of the placebo, and which is reported in more detail in Chapter 4. In the case of pain, at least, the findings have been clear: It has been determined that when placebos are administered, the pain relief is a function of the ability of the placebo to increase the production of the body's own pain relief chemicals—the endorphins or enkephalins. The active mechanism, of course, is the imagination of the recipient. The magic is clearly not in the sugar pill or in the water injection, but rather in the belief attached to them.

Placebo treatment works for problems other than pain, although less is known about the biochemical mechanisms involved. The placebo has been reported to account for healing in from 30% to 70% of all drug and surgical interventions. Even repair of injured tissues has been encouraged with the use of placebo.[10] It no doubt accounts for healing when inappropriate treatments are prescribed, and even for some of the positive effects of appropriate treatment. Placebos, like imagery, hypnosis, and biofeedback, surely must have a direct effect on the immune system, but the components are yet to be carefully researched.

The placebo is actually granting permission to heal; it is a symbol the imagination can incorporate and translate into wondrous biochemical changes that are as yet beyond the comprehension of the finest scientific minds. The wise doctor within each of us knows how to make pain disappear, and tumors melt. It knows whether to call forth T-cells or histamines or endorphins—all in the proper order and combination. The placebo only triggers the process: "Get ready, get set, go!" Surely the time is not far off when we no longer need to provide the artificial stimulus, and the whole process can be begun at will.

According to Jerome Frank, the placebo "gains its potency through being a tangible symbol of the physician's role as healer. In our society, the physician validates his power by prescribing medication, just as a shaman in a primitive tribe may validate his by spitting out a bit of bloodstained down at the proper moment."[7] Hopes and fears, previous experiences, archetypal belief systems, and especially expectancy, all form the basis for the quality and degree of the response.

The effect of the placebo has been well demonstrated in experimental settings, and must be "controlled for" in all drug studies. In other words, when a drug is tested, a group of subjects are given placebos, or fakes that look like the real thing, in order to find out exactly how much of the drug's effectiveness is really in the patient's imagination. In one study, psychiatric patients improved on a number of moods and behaviors as long as they received a capsule. The

ingredients didn't matter; only the capsule was important.[8] The fact
that the placebo effect has been identified in thousands of drug
studies is stark and incontrovertible testimony to the role of the
imagination in health. The wonder is that scientists have invested so
much effort in "controlling" for it, and so little in identifying how it
might be used to best advantage in health care.

The effectiveness of the placebo varies, however, depending
upon how much the patient expects to benefit. For example, Volgyesi,
in 1954, reported on patients who were hospitalized with bleeding
peptic ulcers. They were given water injections and told either (1)
the injections would cure them; or (2) they were being given experimental injections of undetermined effectiveness. Seventy percent of
the first group showed excellent improvement in their conditon,
which was maintained over the follow-up period of one year. Only
25% of the second group showed such improvement.[9]

Even the active properties of drugs can be overcome by the
imagination. Wolf reports on a pregnant woman who, suffering
from morning sickness, was given ipecac and told that it would cure
her nausea. Ipecac is a well-known emetic that is used to produce
vomiting when certain poisons are ingested. It works almost every
time. The woman, however, experienced a cessation of her discomfort, although vomiting and exacerbation of nausea had occurred
when she had taken the drug previously, without these instructions.[10] While some valuable information is gained from this type of
case report, it and many others like it are questionable ethically. The
current trend is to provide complete information on all possible
negative effects, which in itself is problematic, given the propensity
of many patients to expect the worst. A group of oncologists with
whom I spoke is convinced that the required disclosure has increased
side effects of chemotherapy.

And from Norman Cousins, a great journalistic force in moving
the collective attitude of the twentieth century forward toward new
dimensions in health, comes the last word on placebos: "What is
most significant about placebos is not so much the verdict they
supply on the efficacy of new drugs as the clear proof that what
passes through the mind can produce alterations in the body's chemistry. These facts also indicate that the same pathways and connections that come into play through the use of placebos can be activated
without placebos. The main ingredient is the human belief system.
Confidence in the ability to mobilize one's resources is a prodigious
force in itself. The next great advance in human evolution may well

be represented by the ability of humans, working with a new understanding of brain chemistry, to preside over their own beings."[11]

The Imagination in Different Schools of Thought

Theodore X. Barber and other hypnotists claim that the effectiveness
of hypnosis actually lies in the imagery that is created within the
subject by the hypnotic suggestions. Researchers and clinicians,
such as Elmer and Alyce Green, Steve Fahrion and Pat Norris of the
well-established biofeedback laboratory at the Menninger Foundation, acknowledge imagery as a critical element in learning to alter a
physical response through biofeedback training. Schools of psychotherapy and psychological theory, including Gestalt, Psychosynthesis, and Rational Behavior Therapy, depend on imagery to change
behavior, attitude, and health. For all of these, as with shamanic
healing, the ability to change physical or mental function is dependent in the first instance upon the imagery of the patient or healee,
and in the second instance upon the imagination of the therapist.
Rather than doing therapy or treatment or something "to" the patient, the therapists act as guides through the realms of consciousness, suggesting, coaching, using their own inner experience as a
blueprint for the territory.

In the rest of this chapter, I will only touch upon these many
methods. The interested reader will find a vast library available on
them already; others are cited and briefly described in Chapter 5 in
conjunction with social and behavioral science. These different techniques are all paths to the same place. They are all systematic manip-
ulations of the imagination, and they all work for somebody. We
integrate imagery with biofeedback, group therapy, individual counseling, and body work; Larry LeShan uses the imagination with traditional psychotherapy and meditation; and Larry Dossey and other
physicians consciously create imagery through carefully phrased
dialogue with their patients. Joe D. Goldstrich and Dean Ornish use
imagery with nutrition, exercise, and other programs for cardiovascular disease; and Carl and Stephanie Simonton pioneered the
use of imagery with cancer patients in combination with medical
treatment, psychotherapy, and lifestyle change.[12]

The topics that follow are representative of general work going
on within mainline modern medicine. By this, I don't wish to imply
that all these techniques are necessarily accepted by the conservative
allopathic core of medicine, but rather that the practitioners and

practices have an affiliation with mainline medicine, and have either been trained or are functioning within its bounds.

Autogenics

An extensive literature supporting the use of imagery in medicine has been compiled by J. H. Schultz and reported in a seven volume series edited by Wolfgang Luthe.[13] The techniques reported by Schultz and Luthe are collectively known as "autogenic therapy," and are the immediate forerunners of the current application of visualization or guided imagery to health. Careful clinical descriptions of the methods and results are reported for approximately 2,400 cases of every conceivable diagnosis.

Schultz and Luthe employed six standard exercises to be done while patients were sitting or lying in a state of relaxation. The preliminary instructions were to imagine being in mental contact with the parts of the body by centering concentration there, to repeat a special phrase, and to have a casual attitude about the results. The gist of the therapy involved relaxing, imaging the part of the body, and then letting the exercise work instead of trying to force a change (using "passive volition"). These are the major ingredients of all techniques that use the imagination to heal.

The six specific exercises that Schultz and Luthe developed are done in a sequence. First, one is to state over and over, "My right arm is heavy." (The patient might think this silently or be guided by an instructor.) In the second exercise, the task is to imagine feeling warmth in the arms and legs. Then, for the third exercise, the patients continue on to other body systems, viz., "Heart beat calm and regular." The fourth exercise focuses on breathing; the fifth on warming the solar plexus; and the sixth on cooling the forehead. Variations for different maladies are provided. Advanced exercises are complex imagery procedures intended to help gain access to information that is not consciously available.

Autogenic therapy has been documented as successful for both acute and chronic diseases, including asthma, headaches, diabetes, arthritis, low back pain, gastritis, surgical procedures, and dentistry. Physical changes that have been measured include positive effects on muscle potentials, skin temperature, blood sugar, white blood cell counts, blood pressure, heart rate, hormone secretions, and brain waves.

Schultz and Luthe recognized the power of these techniques to heal, if used appropriately; but they were also fully aware of the damage that inappropriate visualizations might cause. For instance, one phrase used in conjunction with relaxation of the abdominal muscles is "my solar plexus is warm." They adamantly state that such a phrase should not be used by persons with gastritis, since those patients are already suffering from increased gastric motility. The increased warmth (which stems from increased blood flow) would in these instances be contraindicated.

Childbirth

Imagery is used systematically to achieve several purposes during childbirth: relaxing, removing fears and anxieties, decreasing pain, sensitizing the mother to the functions of her body, and mentally rehearsing the birth itself. The natural childbirth methods first proposed by English physician Grantly Dick-Read in the 1930s now have many offshoots, all of which are centered around training the mother-to-be to consciously control her physiology and her emotional response to pregnancy and birth. Dick-Read believed the excessive pain associated with childbirth was basically the result of legends of suffering retold from generation to generation. He thought that the pain would be lessened significantly if the fear and the imagery that accompanied the centuries of misrepresentation of the birth process could be cleared.

He began to contradict history by changing the words "uterine pain" to "uterine contraction," and encouraging the fathers to play an active role in delivery. Exercises were developed to be used during labor to relax pelvic musculature. Dick-Read thought fear had a direct effect on the blood flow to the uterus, caused waste products to build up, and activated the sympathetic nervous system. He felt that fear-activated tension could trigger the lower muscles of the uterus into closing against the opening of the cervix, thereby halting or slowing the birth process itself. All in all, he felt that fear directly created an abnormal and excruciating condition.

Dick-Read wanted childbirth to be a more spiritual, conscious occasion for a woman: one that she could fully engage in, while at the same time, not being deprived of the advantages of obstetric medicine. There is now wide acceptance for his methods—even though he was earlier prohibited from practicing them under England's National Health Service. Evidence now exists showing he was absolutely correct in most of his assertions regarding the physical effect of fear.

The second chapter of Dick-Read's classic book, *Childbirth With-*

out Fear, first published in 1942, was devoted to a discussion of the role of imagery. "The memory, or even the visualization of an incident, may surround a natural and physiological function with an aura of pain or pleasure so vivid that normal reflexes are disturbed. . . . Fear of childbirth, then, becomes the great disturber of the neuro-muscular harmony of labor." [14] The message here is clear: If attitudes and images are changed, then the body processes are dramatically affected, and childbirth takes on a whole new perspective.

Russian physicians, using the work of the great physiologist, Ivan Pavlov, approached this premise through his idea of the conditioned response. Responses to stimuli can be learned or conditioned so that they occur with some regularity; but they can also be unlearned. In the case of attitudes toward childbirth, it was believed that if the cultural input of information was changed, the response itself would be altered. The word they used to describe their methods was *psychoprophylaxis*, literally "mental prevention." Essentially, women were taught to mentally dissociate from extreme physical discomfort, and therefore feel it less acutely.

In 1949, the first woman trained in these methods gave birth, attracting the attention of Fernand Lamaze, a French gynecologist. Traveling to Leningrad, he was astounded to see a woman not only awake during the six hours of her labor (those were the days of heavy sedation), but also enjoying it. He took the Russian ideas home with him, modified them, and they spread across Europe and America, later to be known as "Childbirth Without Pain." Lamaze focused his training on teaching women to relax and breathe in very circumscribed ways during the labor and delivery. The breath concentration serves the threefold purpose of physically aiding the birth with an adequate oxygen supply, producing the correct muscular effect during contractions and the interim period between, and also (here's where the psychoprophylaxis comes in), helping the woman mentally dissociate from her discomfort.

One of the modern birthing methods, "Naturebirth," is a combination of the Dick-Read and Lamaze methods, with a feminist, holistic, homeopathic twist and great woman-to-woman appeal. Its founder, Englishwoman Danae Brook, says of the mind prevention aspect of birthing, "the way you breathe is a distraction. Using it you can dissociate from the turbulent activity in your body. If you want to distract yourself as the strongest contractions roll over you, do. Like a meditation technique, this type of breathing gives you a kind of stillness in the eye of the hurricane." Naturebirth training pro-

vides a thorough imaginary rehearsal for the grand event, acquaint-
ing women with their bodies so that they are able to consciously
"single out, feel and control certain muscles, particularly those internal muscles which come into play during labour, but of which few
people are aware during the ordinary course of life before giving
birth."[15] The women also rehearse releasing negative emotions such
as pain, tension, feelings of inhibition and embarrassment. In labor
these only serve to complicate pain and impede progress. Women
practice sitting with their legs flopped open, and grunt and groan
loudly during rehearsal. If anyone complains of indignity, she is
reminded of how absurd it is to feel shame over natural functions.

Mentally rehearsing a feared event in order to lessen its detrimental impact on physiology is one of the most well-documented
aspects of the use of imagery in the medical field. It can be likened
to the rituals of vividly imaging future movements that have been
associated with subsequent peak performance in well-known athletes.[16] Through rehearsal, the body learns to respond in a superb
and automatic fashion when it is time for the actual event.

The sense of transcendence often reported by new mothers who
have actively participated in the birth process, and the athletes' feelings of melding with a timeless cosmos during their finest moments,
are spiritually charged experiences that seem to flow from a common source: preparation through rehearsal. Being prepared allows
one to experience events without unnecessary distraction, and keeps
attention and energy focused. "When your mind and body are being
hurtled into another sense of reality, another dimension, by experience as total as orgasm or birth, the delineations between conscious
and subconscious should go, the physical, feeling self, and the self
which intellectually appraises sensation should be one."[17] For peak
performance, the ego must no longer stand in the way.

The research in support of prepared childbirth for both mother
and child is voluminous. The reduction in the need for pain-killing
medications alone can result in an improved sucking reflex, pulse,
heart and respiratory rate, and generally, in a more healthy and alert
baby and increased mother/child contact. Those of us in the United
States should be particularly concerned about means to enhance the
health of infants, since information gathered by the Statistical Office
of the United Nations shows this country to have an abominable,
inexcusable infant mortality rate. In 1950, the United States was sixth
among industrialized countries, but by 1973 (the most recent official
statistics published), it had dropped to sixteenth—lagging behind

not only the medically advanced Scandinavian countries, but also
Hong Kong, New Zealand, and Canada. Something is wrong.[18]

The world survey conducted in 1973 showed the United States to
have 28.3 infant deaths per 1,000 live births, as compared to the lowest
in Sweden of 9.6. Furthermore, the United States has the highest
rate of infant deaths due to conditions such as postnatal asphyxia
and birth injuries, which are more likely to occur if the mother has
been given pain medication.[19] (According to an independent survey
conducted by Carl Haub, by 1980 the United States had dropped to
nineteenth in terms of infant mortality rates. Actual infant deaths
per 1,000 live births had *decreased*, however, to 12.5.)

Imagery in Nursing

Imagery has found a warm reception among nurses who, as a professional group, are seeking sound clinical tools to accentuate their
identity and independence, as well as to increase the effectiveness of
their practice. In nursing, imagery is likely to be called "sensory
information," although the format used is similar to the guided imagery discussed later in this chapter. Jean Johnson is credited with
giving impetus to the topic through her research. She has gone beyond the boundaries of the customary means of providing patient
education (i.e., talking to patients about the facts of medical procedures), by providing information on the sensory aspects of treatment
as well. Patients are taken on an *a priori* fantasy trip, imaging the particular treatment they are to undergo and what they will experience
with all their senses. People who find themselves requiring medical
care are primarily concerned about what their own personal experience is likely to be, and only secondarily interested in the technical
details of their care. When several studies were made presenting the
sensory aspects to patients about to undergo cholecystectomy, cast
removal, pelvic examination, and endoscopy, the findings were impressive. Individuals who received the sensory information generally
responded better to medical treatment than did the control groups,
even to the extent of significantly decreasing the number of days
spent in the hospital. The patients fared even better when they were
given relaxation instructions prior to the sensory procedure.[20]

Johnson and others who use the sensory information procedure
choose synonyms for words like *pain* whenever possible, and take
care to use words and concepts within the patient's vocabulary.
Johnson also emphasizes the importance of not telling the patients

that the sensory information will reduce their distress or even enable them to cope more effectively.

The sensory information approach offers a modified version of guided imagery, and one that in many respects is more palatable to the standard world of health care than various other imagery techniques. The strategy is designed to help people cope with hospital procedures, and increased coping is always welcomed. The incidental effect on healing time is downplayed, so the medical system is not threatened. The terminology alone will guarantee the would-be practitioner more access to hospitals than words like "healing visualization," "meditation," and "guided imagery," which are still regarded as highly suspect by most physicians.

With sensory information, we once again see not the magic of a procedure, but the potent effect of a prepared mind on a healing body. The effect of mental rehearsal is outstanding, even though expectancy, the most important aspect of healing with the imagination, is deliberately omitted. This, too, makes the approach acceptable to medical professionals, who, as a body, regard the provision of "false hope" as a form of quackery.

Prepared childbirth, sensory information, and guided imagery all have an educational foundation in line with what has been envisioned for the role of medicine. Thomas Edison once said, "The physician of the future will give no medicine, but will interest patients in the care of the human frame, in nutrition, and in the causes and prevention of illness." The word *doctor* itself comes from the Latin *doceo*, "to teach," and only in modern terminology has it come to relate to the practice of prescribing pills and doing surgery.

Imagery and Therapeutic Touch

Drs. Pat Heidt, Gretchen Randolph, and other nurses trained in the use of therapeutic touch have incorporated imagery into their work. "Therapeutic touch" is a kind of scientific laying on of hands developed by Dr. Delores Krieger, who teaches at the Department of Nursing, New York University. The technique has been subjected to numerous experimental analyses and found to be associated with changes in vital signs, blood chemistries, and moderate changes in physical outcome. The research on therapeutic touch does not point to it as a means of effecting lightning-like, dramatic cures, but rather as a stabilizing, relaxing technique that aids in achieving physiological homeostasis.[21]

Of all techniques currently being practiced in medical settings, therapeutic touch is clearly the most aligned with the notion of transpersonal mechanisms of imaginary healing. The practitioners are trained to center their own thoughts, and to be sensitive to receiving and sending nonverbal messages or "energy" through their hands. Blockages that may be the cause or result of disease are identified by changes in "energy field" surrounding the patient. Like imagery, therapeutic touch is intended as a supplemental tool for nurses to use independently in a healing capacity. Too, it is part of the intuitive, noninvasive "soft" medicine that women have practiced forever. Dr. Randolph has integrated therapeutic touch and imagery with a practice of biofeedback, and Dr. Heidt has combined these with her early training as a psychotherapist. The nurses who combine these modalities generally feel there is a synergistic, potentiating effect of one upon the other, particularly since the other techniques enlist the patients' participation. In therapeutic touch the patient is essentially a passive recipient, and the technique is believed to be effective whether or not the patient knows it is taking place.

Dr. Heidt modeled a diagnostic and treatment format after an approach we had developed for cancer patients,[22] and used it in combination with therapeutic touch. She provided her patients with audio tape recordings that contained instructions to help them relax and take a mental journey through their body. They were then asked to draw pictures of their imaginings about their disease or discomfort, how they imagined they could get rid of it, and how their treatment might assist the process. An interview was conducted to explore these themes. In working with patients in a general hospital setting, Heidt found that the imagery served three main functions: (1) It helped her as nurse/investigator to form a close relationship with the patient in a very short period of time; (2) the patients' expression of their feelings about being in the sick role was facilitated; and (3) she was able to learn of the patients' beliefs about their own ability to take part in the healing process—information that is vital to recovery, but not readily obtainable through usual medical histories.[23]

Her experience was that people generally want to tell their stories to health professionals who show an interest in them. "It seems that they want, either consciously or subconsciously, the health professional to understand how they 'see' their own illness and to start the treatment plan from these perceptions."[24]

Imagery in General Medical Practice: Michael Samuels and Irving Oyle

Producing convincing research on the efficacy of using imagery in the general practice of medicine has remained an unmet challenge. First of all, physicians are rarely trained as researchers (the Ph.D., not the M.D., is the research degree), and the few that do have research skills have assiduously avoided the complicated business of mind/body interactions. Furthermore, physicians who are interested in the applications of imagery to clinical practice are busy treating patients, and rarely have either the funds or inclination to pursue research. Government or private foundation money, which would allow physicians to devote time and energy to such study, has never been available. One of the biggest impediments to understanding the effect of the imagination, in and of itself, is that when imagery is used in a general practice, it is rarely employed in isolation from other types of medicine, or even from other nonsurgical, nondrug therapies such as biofeedback. The results of imagery alone are difficult to isolate if the patient is to receive the best possible care, with all appropriate modalities being used.

The failure of the physicians to conduct research on the imagination presents a credibility gap for science and for their peers, but not necessarily for the consumer of health. A horde of popular health materials is available now, written by physicians who have included imagery how-to instructions. Two modern-day physicians, Drs. Irving Oyle and Michael Samuels, write of medicine that incorporates the shamanic tradition. They are not alone, and it is primarily because of their association with general medicine, as opposed to a specialty field, and their accessible, readable books, that I have chosen their work as exemplary. Drs. Dean Ornish, Tom Ferguson, Robert Swearingen, Bernard Siegel, Norman Shealy, Carl Simonton, Joe D. Goldstrich, the many physicians who have attended our workshops and written to us about their use of imagery in their medical practice, and our dear friends, Drs. Larry Dossey, Edmund Tyska, and Rafael Toledo—all of these people, collectively, courageously, are reinstating the role of the imagination, long dethroned.

Michael Samuels, coauthor of *The Well Body Book*, *Seeing with the Mind's Eye*, and *Be Well*, provides a wealth of information on the historical aspects of imagery, as well as application. Trained as a physician at New York University, he worked at San Francisco hospital, on a Hopi Indian Reservation, in a county public health system, and in an holistic clinic. Working with these varied populations, he became dismayed at the lack of understanding people had regarding their own bodies. He believed that, with the proper kind of information, people could largely learn to care for their own health needs. While seeming not to compromise himself on good medical procedure, he has chosen to use imagery as the basic health education and health care tool.

Samuels makes an important distinction between what he calls receptive and programmed visualization, and provides exercises for training in both forms. This is essentially the same distinction that I have made regarding diagnostic versus therapeutic imagery, and describes the two ways that imagery has been used in health for thousands of years. Receptive imagery involves relaxing, tuning in, allowing the spontaneous images to serve diagnostically; while programmed imagery represents the healing component. He states that the latter can be formulated through reading medical, biology, or science textbooks, or even from x-rays or lab tests.

Some of Samuels' general suggestions for healing imagery involve "erasing bacteria or viruses, building new cells to replace damaged ones, making rough areas smooth, making hot areas cool, making sore areas comfortable, making tense areas relax, draining swollen areas, releasing pressure from tight areas, bringing blood to areas that need nutriment or cleansing, making dry areas moist (or moist areas dry), bringing energy to areas that seem tired."[25]

Specific programmed images include the following: For a virus infection, Samuels suggests imagining the viruses as tiny dots on a blackboard, and then erasing the dots. A broken bone or a cut can be imaged as a gap with stones being laid in it by a mason. For a headache, he suggests imagining a hole in your head near the headache and then exhaling the murky, muddy pain through the hole. For an infection of the Fallopian tubes, he advises relaxing the area around the tubes, sensing it as warm and pulsing with energy, and then picturing the tubes themselves as open and draining and lined with pink, healthy mucosa.[26]

The last example of Samuels' work is referred to as a "final-state visualization." This involves visualizing the image of something already healed, which skirts the problems of potential harm that might result from imaging the healing process incorrectly. We must seriously consider this issue: If specific images can result in a corresponding physical change, then damage may also inadvertently occur. (See Appendix A for an example of one of Samuels' visualization exercises.)

Irving Oyle is an osteopathic physician (D.O.), who has been practicing as a family physician for over twenty-five years, and was formerly medical director of the Headlands Healing Service, established in Bolinas, California, in 1971. The service was a project of the Church-World Interaction Committee of the Synod of the Golden Gate United Presbyterian Church. It was intended not only as a prototype experimental community health service for a largely rural population, but also as a place where new techniques of healing could be pioneered. "The operational theory of Headlands Healing Service was to approach the human organism on the physical, psychological and psychic level, believing that, if correctly done, this will effect healing on the physical level."[27] The patients seen by the clinic were evaluated by Dr. Oyle and his staff of physicians with attention to scientific methodology. The records, according to Oyle, are available to interested colleagues.

Oyle states, "All healing is magic. The Indian healer and the western healer have a common denominator. The trust and confidence of both the patient and the healer. They must both believe in the magic or it doesn't work. Western doctors make secret markings on paper and instruct the patient to give it to the oracle in the drug store, make an offering in return for which they will receive a magic potion." Neither, he says, understand exactly how the medicine works, "but if they both believe, it often does."[28]

Realizing that magic comes in many forms, Oyle seems to have tried everything: exorcism, the *I Ching*, sonopuncture (a form of acupuncture using a tuning fork), pyramid power, biofeedback, marijuana, and so forth. He has drawn on the wisdom of Buddhist philosophy, Lao Tzu, Paracelsus, Maharishi Mahesh Yogi, quantum physicists, and Rolling Thunder, the medicine man. Primarily, though, Oyle works with the imagination in ancient ways. His procedures are identical with the incubation sleep techniques practiced by the early Greeks and Christians, and with the shamanic work as well. The patients in each instance are invited into a milieu associated with healing, and encouraged to relax and drift into an altered state of consciousness that is near, but not quite at, sleep. During this state, images come forth that impart the diagnosis, and are sometimes associated with a remarkable cure. (See Appendix B for Oyle's basic imagery exercise.)

One of Oyle's most interesting cases is a woman he calls Lillian, who was diagnosed with nonspecific vaginitis, nonspecific urethritis, and chronic cystitis, meaning that her long-term, perpetual pelvic inflammation and intense burning sensation had no known cause. Lillian began imagining a stream of cool water circulating through her pelvis, and knotted ropes being untied. What felt like a cement block in her lower back was imaged as dissolving. She said she felt better; the burning was still there, but covered a smaller area.

Then, one night when Lillian was practicing her imagery at home, a coyote named Wildwood flashed into her mind. He advised her to stay by his side, and watch what was about to happen, and told her that what she saw would be related to the fire in her body. She then sensed herself sitting by a campfire, in the midst of a hostile tribe of Indians who held her captive. She experienced the horror of being brutally gang-raped and murdered. "At the instant of my death . . . I woke up and was back in my body in my room, only my pain was completely gone, and hasn't returned since."[29] Oyle's patient chose to attribute her experience to a past life, even though she'd never believed in reincarnation previously. Whatever the explanation, her own imagination had worked powerfully to both diagnose and cure her disease.

When the imagination works so dramatically for general medical conditions, professionals steeped in modern technology and medicine and twentieth-century psychology usually feel impelled to come up with an acceptable explanation. Either they decide the illness was probably all in the patient's head to begin with (i.e., he/she was either hysterical or hypochondriacal or both), or that some dammed up energy (usually of a sexual nature) had been released as a result of therapy. Three other common explanations for unusual recovery are: (1) the medicines finally took effect; (2) it was just time for it to go away, and the imagery was coincidental; (3) the patient had been misdiagnosed. Oyle's methods and results are not uncommon among the new shaman/scientists' findings. When we cling to the more "rational" explanations of such cures, we have lost sight of our ancient roots, and may well be ignoring some contemporary facts.

Biofeedback: Self as Shaman?

In 1975, an article appeared in the *Journal of the American Medical Association* that referred to the *"furor therapeuticus"* that had arisen about a "field of research whose clinical applications are still uncertain, but that has raised dazzling prospects for healing."[30] Since that time, biofeedback, the field in question, has become one of the most credible behavioral techniques designed for medical application. For disorders such as migraine and tension headache, gastrointestinal problems, Raynaud's syndrome, chronic pain, for rehabilitation following stroke and injuries, and for prevention and alleviation of many stress-related problems, it is no longer regarded as an experimental procedure.

Encouraging results have been published that support the role of biofeedback in the treatment of numerous other conditions, including arthritis, diabetes, cardiovascular disease (especially hypertension), speech disorders, and tinnitus, to mention but a few. The research base is extensive. Biofeedback is even more thoroughly documented and studied than most medical protocols, including drugs and surgical procedures. Of all the imagery healing techniques mentioned in this book, it is the only one reimbursed by major medical insurance companies.

Biofeedback generally refers to any technique that uses instrumentation to provide signals of bodily function. As such, both scales and mirrors might be considered biofeedback. Normally, though, technical biofeedback implies the use of sophisticated instruments that can accurately measure and rapidly provide feedback in ongoing levels of brain wave activity, muscle firing, blood flow and skin temperature, heart rate, blood pressure, and so forth. The clinical importance of biofeedback is that once the level and minute changes in these functions are known, *they can be brought under conscious control.* To date, there is evidence that every physical function that can be measured in this way can be controlled or regulated to some extent. The implications for the practice of medicine are tremendous, and only the surface of the potential of biofeedback has been scratched.[31]

It should be evident by now that human beings did not have to wait upon the innovations of modern technology to learn to alter their physiology. Yogis and shamans have been doing it forever, but only after serious concentration and years of quiet, inner focusing. As a consequence of their discipline, they are able to achieve exquisite attunement to internal events, and attain control over them. Biofeedback instrumentation merely makes the process more efficient.

The clinical aspects of biofeedback require that the person learn to do "something" with the mind that allows conscious communication with the body. This "something" does not relate to words, but to images engaging the various sensory and motor systems (the visual and auditory systems, kinesthesis, and touch, for example). The images, as we will describe in Chapter 4, are the language the body understands, particularly with regard to the autonomic or involuntary nervous system. The biofeedback instruments are designed to inform the patient of whether or not the image has had the desired effect, i.e., whether temperature has gone up or down, muscle tension has changed, or brain waves altered. Feedback is critical for any kind of learning to occur. Without feedback on whether the performance has been correct or not, we would never learn to ride a bike or work a math problem, much less consciously change our physiology.

Biofeedback involves healing in the imaginary realms, and fits well within the rubric of preverbal healing using the imagination. It contains aspects of shamanism: Rituals are conducted, the subject goes into an altered state of consciousness, takes an imaginary journey, and enters into a territory where healing information is available. In the case of biofeedback, however, the journey is ostensibly inward, and not out to the upperworld and the underworld of the shaman.

As technology enters into the terrain of imaginary healing, however, shamanism takes on a new perspective. Since ancient times, those who exercised their potential for healing others with the imagination (i.e., transpersonal healing) were a few hardy souls who braved pain and danger and dedicated their lives to the endeavor. Now it appears that with new knowledge of the body/mind communication system and proper teaching, such as the electronic gadgetry promises, we can all eventually learn to enter an altered state of consciousness at will and exercise our own healing mechanisms. Shamanism, as it has been practiced in the traditional manner of healing, may become obsolete after 20,000 years.

Not everyone responds well to biofeedback therapy, and an examination of the reasons for those failures points to human, not technological, problems. The best success rates across all diagnoses average around sixty percent. The clinics and laboratories that report these results typically use well-trained clinicians and a combination of biofeedback, patient education, and meditation. Just hooking someone up to a machine doesn't work. Like the shaman, the therapist or clinician must have traveled through his/her own imaginary landscapes in order to teach the route that is without words.

In examining the characteristics of people who don't respond to biofeedback, we encounter some common findings. Biofeedback requires the persistent involvement of highly motivated persons, who are able and willing to spend time and effort on their own health. It is neither easy nor cheap. It requires a belief that it will work and trust in the practitioner. Beyond these motivational issues, the ability to learn to consciously regulate physiology appears to vary across the population like any other human trait, with some people naturally very able, and others who have extreme difficulty in performing the task.

In a recent study, we attempted to identify the basis for individual differences in learning biofeedback, and it appeared to be the ability to use the imagination.[32] Those individuals who were unable to fantasize, who seldom remembered their dreams, and who were not regarded as particularly creative, had the most difficulty in learning the biofeedback response. These findings were incidental to the purpose of the study, which was to compare biofeedback with the usual physical therapy modalities, using a group of women diagnosed with rheumatoid arthritis. Biofeedback was used primarily to train these women to relax. The biofeedback group was highly successful on measures related to decreases in pain, anxiety, and sleep problems. The most encouraging findings came from a blood analysis used to measure disease activity, called sedimentation rate. All of the biofeedback subjects' blood tests had returned to normal, nondiseased levels by the end of the study.

The best results, however, were obtained from those women who were able to use their imaginations—particularly as it related to imaging the desired health outcome. This, as well as results from the field in general, points to the conclusion that the function of biofeedback is actually to teach the imagination, with the outcome being communication to body systems via the imaginary paths. Techniques for directly working with the imagery modality follow.

Imagery as a Diagnostic and Therapeutic Tool

Dr. G. Frank Lawlis and I have researched and practiced imagery in a variety of health care settings over the past decade. Imagery, as we use it, combines twentieth-century understanding of health and disease with ancient shamanic techniques. We call our technique bodymind imagery. It has been validated on patients having chronic pain, rheumatoid arthritis, cancer, diabetes, severe orthopedic trauma, burn injury, alcoholism, and stress-related disorders such as migraine headaches and hypertension, and during childbirth. The work has been published in professional journals, presented to colleagues in professional forums, and has served as the topic of numerous unpublished doctoral dissertations. The research base, together with an emphasis on physiology, distinguishes the bodymind imagery from other approaches. It was developed out of the belief that the shamanic techniques that served the world so well as medicine since the beginning of recorded history should not be discarded, but improved upon.

General guidelines for using imagery in both diagnosis and therapy are provided below. Following that, the application of body-mind imagery as mental rehearsal will be discussed.[33]

Preparation for Use of Imagery as a Healing Tool

We advise the would-be imagery practitioner (both patient and therapist) to begin by developing a solid understanding of the way the body functions, and by gathering information on the health condition under concern. Physiology, neuroanatomy and gross anatomy can be learned through the aid of a number of self-help books on the market, and medical information is available in textbooks and in medical journals. These are quite comprehensible, once the jargon and format are understood. Bookstores are full of health-related materials, and foundations (such as the support groups for major diseases) are generous with their information.

It is important to stay current with treatment methods and thoroughly research any treatment that might be underway. This assures that the patient is a knowledgeable and willing participant, capable of making judgments on his/her own behalf. Medications can be checked out in terms of treatment implications and possible problems in usage in the *Physician's Desk Reference* (*PDR*). How effective is the drug supposed to be? This is a difficult question, and takes much sleuthing beyond the drug salesperson's claims and into the actual material of the scientific trials. One must be wary here; drug trials are paid for by the companies who manufacture the drugs; and, although most claim to be scrupulous, there have been problems. It is helpful if the patients learn something, regardless of how simple, about how the pills work, and, if surgery is to be undertaken, how it is supposed to cure the problem. All this information aids the image formation significantly, and is intended to enhance that all-important belief system—not to harass the doctor.

For the therapist, understanding the dimensions of the diseases of his patients is crucial for the application of imagery. The cancer patient faces unique circumstances in living compared to the person with myocardial infarction—and current research indicates they may have had different kinds of personalities prior to their diagnosis. Knowledge of odds for survival and propensity for recovery guide the therapeutic interaction. When the balance is not in favor, the fight must be harder, but not necessarily viewed with more hopelessness. Image programming should be realistic in this respect. There are some things bodies and minds just don't know how to heal yet, and which modern medicine can't help either, such as spinal cord injury, or the progressive and irreversible deterioration of major organs that can't be replaced with any degree of success. More often though, the potential of recovery from major diseases is underplayed. Roughly one-third or more of all cancer patients, rheumatoid arthritics, not to mention those with such plagues as ulcers, asthma, and even schizophrenia, will undergo remissions. Hope and belief in becoming one of the positive health statistics stir the imagination into action.

The most useful information on disease has come from those people who have been diagnosed with a condition and can articulate how they have mastered it or learned to live a fulfilling life in spite of it. We ask them especially about the details of the actual healing: what it felt like, and what sensations, thoughts or behaviors accompanied or preceded the healing process. My patients have told me fascinating things in this regard, usually having something to do with special mental activity.

I'm reminded of a young man who was working on a scaffold when a crane swung into it, sending him hurtling down two stories. His arm was nearly severed, he broke both of his knees, sustained multiple fractures, and injured his back. There was no logical reason for him to have survived, except that he's mentally as tough as nails. When I asked him how he did it, he said he knew he had to keep his eyes open, because if he became unconscious, he'd never wake up again. He remained awake throughout the ordeal, watching the blood and "white stuff" flow out of his arm, acutely aware of the pain, and never going into shock. He focused on his breathing, holding his breath as long as he could and then breathing shallowly. A fellow construction worker helped save his arm by applying pressure in the right places. After hours and hours of careful surgery, it was successfully reattached, and has now become functional. He still fights general anesthesia and every other situation where he might lose the self-control that pulled him through. He holds his breath, and steels himself for his next life crisis; but he's alive.

Stories of spectacular, unexpected recovery often include a description of extreme heat, tingling, numbness, or itching in the area of the disease—all compatible with an enhanced immune response. Sometimes the first clue that a disease is going away comes in a dream, or in a state of reverie. A kind of "knowing" is described that accompanies a successful treatment (and I am using the word *treat-*

ment here to include nonmedical procedures such as religious experience, vitamins, exercise, and meditation). The treatment is often said to lead to a sense of calm and diffused warmth and comfort as the disease is released. People describe images of being filled with white light, or of seeing an incandescent globe hover over their bodies right before they have the sense of being healed. Patients who recover quickly from surgery often talk about having done significant mental work while lying in bed, assisting the healing process with their imaginations. A nurse who was injured on the ski slopes imaged her fractures being bridged by new bone, for instance, and even surprised herself at her rate of recovery.

When patients tell their stories and describe their imagery, it normally involves more information on what it's like to be sick than on how they got well, or managed to keep themselves alive. This anchors us in the world of pain and fear and uncertainty, but beyond a point, becomes nonproductive as far as learning to create positive imagery for health.

Imagery as Diagnosis

Throughout the history of medicine, including the shamanic healing traditions, the Greek tradition of Asclepius, Aristotle and Hippocrates, and the folk and religious healers, the imagination has been used to diagnose disease. Our imagery procedures follow that lead.

First of all, it is necessary to learn to relax deeply beforehand so motor responses, thoughts and external stimuli don't compete with the production of imagery. The Jacobsen method of relaxation (tensing and relaxing each muscle) is notably ineffective for imagery induction. (The relaxation script that I use appears in Appendix C.) About any type of relaxation will do, provided it doesn't take more than twenty minutes, and isn't too full of words; too much verbal content keeps the left brain actively competing for attention. All of the healing traditions employ this critical first step, some with more ritual than others.

The setting is important: It, as well as the ritual, should be designed to increase belief, not anxiety. More often than not the setting is that of a hospital, clinic, or a biofeedback laboratory. These places are the healing shrines of modern civilization, and tend to have power and expectancy associated with them. In some instances, I recommend seeking out a natural healing place—a place of power, as the Indian healers would say: the peace of the desert or the cleansing ferment of the ocean or the rarefied air and beauty of the mountains. Spending several hours or days in quiet contemplation, using fire or candles or crystals to intensify concentration, listening to drum beats or special music—all these are ways humans manage to carry themselves to the depths of consciousness. The images that are important for health seem to arise close to the point of sleep, but also during the dream state. (A script for taking a mental journey to identify the components of disease and to identify personal defenses appears in Appendix D).

Assessment of Images

The therapist's goal at this point is to create a canvas upon which the intimate knowledge of disease can then be drawn, but not to program or suggest images. It is upon the initial hunches, the emotions, the strength given to the disease and the defenses rallied against it that therapy is based.

Since preverbal imagery is involved, assessment is aided by eliminating words as much as possible in the therapeutic interaction. To help with this, we ask the patients to draw the three major components of the imagery: the disease, the treatment, and the defenses. The images are then examined and evaluated in the following ways:

(1) the disease imagery is assessed for the vividness of the image, its strength (or weakness), and its ability to persist;

(2) the treatment imagery is examined for vividness and effectiveness of the mechanism for cure; and

(3) the imagery for personal defenses is evaluated in terms of the vividness of their description, and the effectiveness of their action.

The overall coherence of the three components, how well the story is integrated, and the degree of symbolism have also proved to be important. The more symbolic images, as opposed to those that are realistic or anatomically correct, are better predictors of good health outcome.[34]

Some questions asked of the imagery might be: How well is the person coping with the disease? Is the seriousness of the disease being denied? Are the images consistent with medical facts? Who's winning—the disease, treatment, or host defenses? Who or what does this person believe could be ultimately responsible for any healing that takes place? How indicative is the imagery of good outcome? When the statistical tests aren't used, the answers require common sense and a knowledge of the significance and meaning the person attaches to the images.

Using images from the reverie or dream state to diagnose ailments has consistently required shamanic wisdom. In Chapters 1 and 2, many examples were given of the ways images were induced and used to diagnose throughout the history of medicine. Usually, though, diagnosis went beyond purely assessing the physical aspects of the disease. Diagnosis encompassed, as well, understanding the disease in both a cultural and individual context, determining why the person had lost "power" and allowed the disease to enter in the first place, and looking for spiritual crisis. We have attempted to combine these pivotal aspects of shamanic healing with current concepts of health.

For example, after the diagnostic imagery is considered, the meaning of both the disease and the symbols used to describe the disease and the defenses against it can be addressed. Diseases have taken on idiosyncratic cultural meaning and they are each person's unique response to his or her lifestyle. We inquire about what might have caused life to lose meaning, what situations were encountered that stressed a person beyond his/her limits (i.e., why he/she lost "power"), and look for an interpretation of the problems within the patient's spiritual system of belief. Disease, especially serious disease, provokes more thought about the meaning and purpose of life than any other event, and deserves to be explored in that regard. These are significant omissions in the way medicine is usually practiced today.

Imagery as Therapy

The discussion of the diagnostic imagery serves as the beginning of the therapy procedure. This can be a very enlightening experience in terms of understanding the meaning of the disease from a patient's perspective. The images of treatment, for example, may be grossly incorrect or just blurry. The idea of personal defenses may be a new one, and require education about their nature. The images should be consonant with fact, even if those facts are symbolized. One patient with rheumatoid arthritis had read about cancer patients who imaged their white blood cells as white knights. Deciding that would be good for her, too, she began imaging up whole battalions to kill her arthritis. Rheumatoid arthritis, an autoimmune disorder, would be significantly worsened by hyperactive white blood cells such as she had envisioned. Persons with diabetes often image the high blood sugar as their problem, and imagine that it will be solved if the blood sugar would just leave. In truth, their primary problem is that the mechanism for transporting sugar into the cells and metabolizing it for food is deficient; hence it stays in the blood stream. So disease education fits in readily at this stage of the imagery training. Understanding the disease is often the beginning of cure. Pictures from textbooks, journals, drug advertisements and anatomy models are all helpful, and I have found a few artists who are able to translate difficult material into simple drawings conducive to image formation.

Following this exploration, suggestions are given on how to revamp the imagery so that it conforms with what is known about the human body, and then on how to create an imaginary situation where the disease is released through both treatment and natural mechanism. The persons who use the imagination to successfully achieve health put considerable mental energy into this process. They take it seriously, spending at least thirty minutes a day exclusively in mental healing. Always, the relaxation must come first, followed by the image work. Most people experience definite sensations in whatever area they are concentrating upon. They "try on" images until they find ones that fit, and they describe spontaneous changes in images, which often foretell important physical changes. They image while they jog, and while waiting at stop lights.

The kind of imagery I've just described alters body function and changes attitudes for all the reasons that will be discussed in Chapters 4 to 6. It appeals to the sense of taking charge and gaining control over physiology. It could be conceived of only after the brilliant discoveries of contemporary science and medicine; and, at the same time, it is impeded by our failure to understand the details of what triggers the body to heal itself. However, imagery that takes into consideration what is known about physiology can be said to become a ritual that incorporates the values of a modern age.

Imagery as Mental Rehearsal

The idea of mentally rehearsing painful or anxiety-laden events is one of the most acceptable uses of imagery in the modern health practice. As discussed previously, it forms the basis for natural childbirth methods. Mental rehearsal also can be given credit for the positive effects on health observed in patients whose education includes imaginary journeys through fearful diagnostic and treatment procedures.

The physical effects of mental rehearsal have been well documented with athletes, particularly. Kiester describes how runner James Robinson mentally rehearsed every split second of the 800 meters he would run in the Olympics, down to "the hiss of his breath and the crunch under his feet,"[35] hoping it would mean the difference between first and second place. Robert Nideffer, a sports psychologist at the Olympic training camp, advised not only using imagery and visualization, but staying in touch with feelings and emotions and mentally rehearsing every split second in "real time." World champion diver Greg Louganis visualizes his dives and coordinates each of his moves to music, going over kinesthetic and visual cues. Dennis Golden, chairman of the Sports Science Committee for Diving, shows his divers video tapes again and again, until the visualization becomes second nature.

The benefits of the imagery techniques described above are many. The athletes learn to overcome anxieties and self-doubts, and actually go through a subtle muscular workout that facilitates coordination and peak performance. Furthermore, they are training themselves to function automatically and to become desensitized to emotions and other distractions that would inhibit their performance.

People whose bodies are being challenged by illness and treatment might well be compared to athletes facing championship competition. They will need to call forth all the physical and mental resources they can muster. Usually the pain involved is significantly complicated and exacerbated by anxiety. Courage, fortitude, and the ability to face the unknown will all be required. Nowhere is this more apparent than on the burn unit.

For the past three years, Cornelia Kenner and I have studied the effect of imagery used as mental rehearsal on patients with major burn injuries.[36] The individuals we worked with experienced more pain than most of us can imagine being humanly possible. During and immediately following the burn, they tended to mentally dissociate, often claiming their minds bounced up to the ceiling, allowing them to dispassionately view what was going on below. It is the treatment, not the burn itself, that most recall as being practically unendurable. In the burn unit where we conducted the research, the treatment involved going to the tanks or showers at least once a day and having the devitalized skin removed or debrided. Usually this was done without the benefit of painkillers, so the patients weren't groggy and could help get themselves to and from the procedures. Sometimes it went on for months, depending upon the size of the burn. It was frequently described as feeling like being skinned alive.

Prior to beginning the study, we followed many patients through their treatment, monitored their physiology, and talked to them about their experiences. We noted that the temperature of their hands and feet would drop twenty degrees within five minutes after they heard the instrument cart come down the hall. (The cart was pushed by a technician or nurse, and contained the instruments for cutting off their bandages. This was the first step in the debridement procedure.) This much of a temperature drop indicates a severe flight or fight response, or a rapid activation of the sympathetic nervous system (see Chapter 4). Also, the blood pressure, respiration, and heart rate increased significantly.

After their old bandages were removed (a painful procedure, since they stick to the skin), all but the most severely and newly burned were required to walk down the hall to the tanks and showers. Many of the patients had burns over 50% and more of their bodies, so the walk itself was difficult, but necessary, since significant problems with blood clots can occur when people stay in bed for long periods. After entering the water, the patients were scrubbed with rough brushes, and large pieces of skin were removed with tweezers. After the patients returned to their beds, they often had to wait unclothed and uncovered for fifteen minutes to an hour while the doctors, medical students, physical therapists, social workers, etc., made their rounds. The body's natural response in such a situation is intense shivering to help restore warmth. The indignities suffered in these open wards goes without saying. But there was a secondary factor of not knowing what new treatment would be recommended during rounds: grafting, amputation, plastic surgery, or a stepped-up program of painful physical therapy were all possible. After the rounds came a tranquil time, when soothing antibiotic cream was spread on their burns, and fresh bandages were put on.

The patients were faced with a situation of the most acute pain imaginable. Also, the fear level was understandably intense and unremitting. The Institute of Nursing, National Institute of Health, in Washington, D.C., agreed with our proposal to develop methods of pain and anxiety control that could later be applied by other nursing staffs on burn units. We were funded for three years. During that time, we tested three methods of pain and anxiety control and compared them with a no-treatment control group (to make sure that attention was not a factor in any results obtained). The methods chosen were: (1) relaxation; (2) a combination of relaxation and imagery; and (3) a program of relaxation, imagery and biofeedback combined. Because the relaxation and imagery combination was the most successful, and most central to the theme of this writing, I will focus upon it primarily.

We studied 149 patients in the four groups. The average percentage of body area burned was 25%. Most had mixed second and third degree burns. The measures we chose to determine success of the methods included vital signs (heart rate, respiration, and blood pressure), the patients' own estimate of pain, a standardized measure of anxiety, the amounts of pain medication, tranquilizers, and sleep medication they required, muscle tension (EMG recordings), and peripheral temperature (another anxiety measure).

The patients were assigned to groups, then trained either in one of the three treatment regimens, or, if they were assigned to the control group, they were just observed and their responses measured. All the patients were given only three training sessions, because we had to move quickly before their debridement procedure was prescribed (usually a few days after the burn injury). Then, prior to the debridement, the treatment regimen was administered. Again, the intention was to reduce some of the pain/anxiety complex before, during and after the debridement.

Neither the control group nor the relaxation group showed any benefit. Both other groups benefited according to measures of reduced anxiety and pain, but the addition of the biofeedback was not particularly useful, and with some measures, the relaxation and imagery combination was better. For example, the group that received relaxation and imagery had less muscle tension, and required significantly fewer pain medications and sedatives than did the group that had biofeedback added to the combination. We interpreted this to mean that during acutely painful states, it is not so important to get in touch with and control body functions (the purpose of biofeedback), but rather to learn mental techniques for dealing with the stressful situations.

The imagery used was intended to be a mental rehearsal for the debridement procedures, one that would inform, desensitize, reduce anxiety, and provide helpful suggestions on relaxing and using the mind to escape the difficult times. All information was audio taped in my voice, and was administered by research technicians, who also collected the data. (The script used appears in Appendix E.)

This complex study, with its several groups and many measures, can be summarized succinctly. It demonstrated the efficacy of behavioral methods in the management of acute pain and anxiety, with mental rehearsal or imagery being the most successful. In many ways, the results were surprisingly good, given the circumstances. Our research technicians were not trained as therapists, the turnover of personnel was considerable because of the stress of working on the burn unit, and the research design prohibited tailoring treatment to an individual's special needs. Also, tape recordings were the primary mode of therapy, and one would expect they would be inferior to personal induction. Nevertheless, given this minimum guidance, the patients were able to significantly reduce their discomfort—another triumph for the human psyche.

Conclusion

In summary, healing with the gifts of the imagination, long the province of the shaman, has taken an extraordinary new direction. No longer are these talents considered the exclusive territory of a privileged few; now they are accessible to all as a function of developments in science, technology, and innovations in medical practice. The common element in each of the techniques discussed in this chapter is the active participation of the patient. In the modern health setting, the healee also becomes the healer, while the shaman dons the role of teacher.

The techniques that incorporate both science and shamanism neither require nor negate the assumptions of the transpersonal mode of healing with the imagination; i.e., the assumption that the consciousness of one person can positively affect the health of another through unknown channels of information transfer. It is also unnecessary to ascribe to a spiritual interpretation of how healing takes place in order to make these techniques work. The explanatory mechanisms (such as those described in subsequent chapters) substantiate the preverbal concept of imaginary healing.

Despite the critical differences between the basic assumptions underlying the traditional shamanic practice and the techniques of the shaman/scientist, there are similarities. Both the shaman and the shaman/scientist rely on common elements to create health: an atmosphere of trust and expectancy, an understanding of the meaning of disease in both a social and personal context, and the use of culturally sanctioned rituals and symbols. (See Chapter 5 for a more complete discussion of these issues.) What has been lost in terms of the mystery of the shaman's power to heal (and mystery does indeed have power) has surely been redeemed by the addition of scientific knowledge.

I should add a final reminder to this topic: Throughout this book I have focused on only a circumscribed aspect of shamanic work—healing with the imagination. The shamans use several other methods of healing, and often serve as political, economic, and spiritual leaders. The data supporting the work of the shaman/scientist in health, while perhaps relevant, is by no means addressed to these additional roles.

4 Science and the Imagination: Physiology and Biochemistry

> The brain is an enchanted loom, weaving a dissolving pattern, always a meaningful pattern, though never an abiding one, a shifting harmony of subpatterns.
>
> *C. S. Sherrington, 1940*

Having discussed the forms that healing with the imagination has taken past and present, in the next section of the book I will present the scientific evidence for how this might work. Claude Bernard, the renowned founder of experimental medicine, advised that the appropriate study of physiology consisted of taking the complex manifestations of the organism, reducing them to simple properties, and then reconstructing the whole by uniting the "elementary relations." Following his advice, in this chapter I will briefly review the psychophysiological aspects of imagery, and then describe the structure and function of the central nervous system (CNS) as they relate to the thesis at hand, i.e., the role of the imagination in health. Then, the relationship among the constituencies of the CNS will be mapped. Last, the holographic model of brain function proposed by Karl Pribram will be used to account for what's left over when the function of the whole cannot be accounted for by adding up the parts.

Imagining Makes It Happen

The initial proposition here is that images affect physical reactions directly and indirectly, and, in turn, are affected by those reactions.

The images may involve any sensory system, but can just as well occur in the absence of the appropriate external stimulation (i.e., light waves, sound waves, molecules of odor). The images are believed to generate similar, but not necessarily identical, internal response states as the actual stimuli themselves. For instance, during visualization experiences, the visual cortex is normally activated, but the more peripheral visual pathways such as the pupil may or may not be involved. Some investigators even suggest that the imagery is coded in special ways and transcends most of the sensory pathways altogether.[1]

Physiology
Physiological Correlates of the Image

People who experience very intensive imagery may have full-blown physiological responses. These "eidetikers," as they are called, are able to recall past events in minute detail, as if their memory storage banks weren't at all muddied up by time or feelings. One of the most famous cases, reported by Alexander Luria, was a man who was able to increase his heart rate by imagining himself running, and who could alter the size of his pupils and manipulate his cochlear reflex by imaging sights and sounds.[2]

In 1929, Jacobsen demonstrated that if one thinks intensively about a particular body movement, the appropriate motor neurons are activated. To be sure, the rate of firing is extremely low, and muscle activity is perceptible only with sensitive recording instruments. Nevertheless, thinking about swinging a golf club actually triggers those muscles to become active. The swing is rehearsed and perfected in just this fashion—a well-established practice among professional athletes. Imagining eating a lemon, or just thinking of increasing the amount of saliva, has a direct effect on the production of the salivary glands.[3]

Intensive sexual and phobic imagery is accompanied by dramatic physiological changes.[4] Imaging noxious stimuli has been associated with physiological arousal as measured by heart rate, muscle tension, and skin resistance levels.[5] In an early study in this area, subjects were instructed to image lifting different weights. Muscle tension increased according to the heft suggested by the experimenter, and very vivid images were related to more muscle tension.[6] Work by Barber suggests that images can elicit changes in blood glucose, gastrointestinal activity, and blister formation.[7] Pioneering investigations by Schneider and Smith and their colleagues, and Hall have determined that the image is also capable of controlling aspects of the immune system.[8]

Imagining oneself in a pleasant, nonthreatening scene is a commonly used method for slowing down a pounding heart, lowering blood pressure, and generally achieving a homeostatic balance. Desensitization, a popular method of dealing with significant and maladaptive fears and anxieties, relies on the use of imagery in this regard: Unpleasant events are imagined during deep relaxation, thus conditioning those thoughts to a state of calmness, and "unlearning" the association between them and a high level of physiological arousal. Desensitization is believed to work because it is theoretically impossible to feel either fear or anxiety while physically relaxed. The hundreds of reports on this technique make it one of the most extensively tested and documented therapeutic approaches, and a testimony to the role of the imagination in determining behavior.[9]

Other findings of consequence in understanding how images are intricately involved in behavior, attitudes, and physical change include those of Jordan and Lenington. They demonstrated that intensive images of negative childhood memories are accompanied by changes in heart rate, galvanic skin response, respiration, and eye movement.[10] Gary Schwartz and his colleagues found that imagery associated with sadness, anger, and fear could be differentiated by cardiovascular changes.[11]

Taken together, the studies demonstrate that images have a direct effect on the body. The effect of the image has been noted not only on the musculoskeletal system, but on the autonomic or involuntary nervous system as well. Certain of the changes evoked by the image (heart rate, muscle changes) might be attributable to either respiratory or skeletal maneuvers normally amenable to conscious control. Other responses, such as increased salivation, changes in the immune system, skin and vascular changes, appear to be accessed directly by the image via the autonomic nervous system.

The general research findings on imagery and physiology are as follows:

(1) Images relate to physiological states;

(2) Images may either precede or follow physiological changes, indicating both a causative and reactive role;

(3) Images can be induced by conscious, deliberate behaviors, as well as by subconscious acts (electrical stimulation of the brain, reverie, dreaming, etc.);

(4) Images can be considered as the hypothetical bridge

between conscious processing of information and physiological change;

(5) Images can exhibit influence over the voluntary (peripheral) nervous system, as well as the involuntary (autonomic) nervous system.

Overview of the Nervous System

Our understanding of how the human brain functions has come essentially from the study of damaged brains: brains that were diseased from tumors or stroke, or brains that had been shot at, cut into, or were congenitally abnormal. Other information has been gleaned from the animal lab, where deliberate changes in the brain are created either by selective damage, stimulation with electricity, or chemicals. These methods of studying the role and function of various structures naturally leave the findings open to criticism as to their relevancy for the normal or nondamaged human brain. Even so, neither technology nor human ethics has come forth with any more acceptable solution to the quest for information on the human brain.

There is a new generation of technology that includes placing recording electrodes—often hundreds—in multiple locations in the brain, and using chemical tracer techniques that will literally monitor the transmission of thought. When these techniques are trained on the subject of the imagination, we will burst into a new era of discovery. Nevertheless, by tying together the existing research, it is possible to construct a theoretical framework supporting the role of imagination as the link between thought and physical change.

Before the route of the image from brain to behavior is traced, the following is offered as a quick review of the nervous system.

The nervous system is arbitrarily divided into two major components: the *central nervous system* and the *peripheral nervous system*. (See Figure 4-1 for a schematic of these divisions.) The central nervous system is then subdivided into its two major components, the *brain* and the *spinal cord*. The cord conducts impulses to and from the brain, and is the only route to the brain from the rest of the body.

The brain is composed of approximately a hundred billion to a trillion neurons, or nerve cells, imbedded in a supportive network of glial cells. The glial cells form the neurons' only access to the nutrients from the blood, and they act to filter, synthesize, and store materials for use by the neurons. The three divisions of the brain are *forebrain, midbrain,* and *hindbrain*. The forebrain consists of the *telen-*

cephalon and *diencephalon*. The telecephalon areas with which we will be concerned here are the *cerebral cortex* and the *limbic system*. The diencephalon includes the *thalamus*, the *hypothalamus*, and the *pituitary*, among other things. The midbrain contains both *visual* and *auditory pathways*, and areas related to muscular control. The hindbrain contains the *cerebellum*, the *pons*, and the *medulla oblongata*—areas that are rich in neural pathways.

The peripheral nervous system consists of the *somatic nervous system* (SNS) and the *autonomic nervous system* (ANS). The SNS has twelve pairs of *cranial nerves* and thirty-one pairs of *spinal nerves*. The function of this branch is to maintain contact with the outside world. It delivers impulses from the central nervous system to striated muscles, and very discreet types of voluntary action are then possible. The ANS was believed to be involuntary and beyond conscious control. Now we know that is only partially true. The heart, liver, spleen, pancreas, intestines, blood vessels, glands, and the urogenital system are all influenced by the ANS, and hence, within reach of conscious determination.

The ANS is generally responsible for the maintenance of the internal environment, whereas the SNS is involved in reacting to stimuli of the external world. We have a ready-made physiological dualism that conforms to the notion of a higher (i.e., cortical) control versus a lower (subcortical, or more primitive) control. This, of course, is a grossly oversimplified, but not incorrect, conceptualization that will help explain the imagery pathways.

The ANS can be divided into two systems—the *sympathetic* and the *parasympathetic*. While there is great overlap in the function of these two systems, the sympathetic branch can be thought of as taking over when action is needed, and the parasympathetic when balance or homeostasis is required. Both systems are activated by releasing factors manufactured in the hypothalamus. These, in turn signal the production and release of hormones in the pituitary gland, and subsequently, the secretion of all the endocrine glands.

Transmission of Information

Information in the central nervous system is carried from one structure to another via fiber tracts or bundles of neurons, whose properties are electrochemical in nature. Think of the neuron as a bag of fluid that has an information receiving area (the *dendrites*), and an information sending area (the *axon*)—often a long, filamentous snaky-looking affair. A neuron "fires" or becomes active when the dendrites

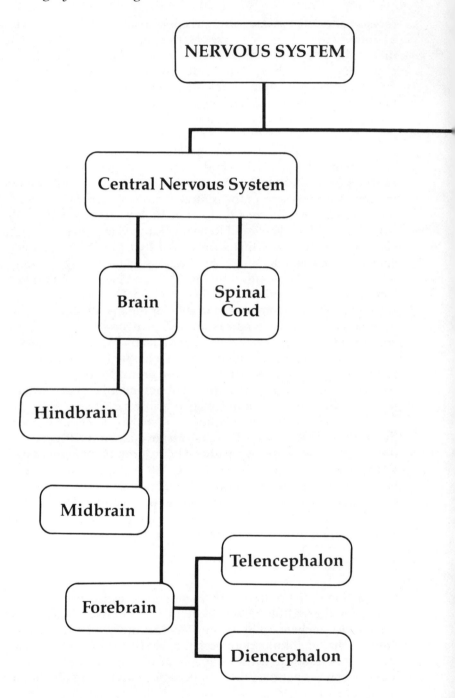

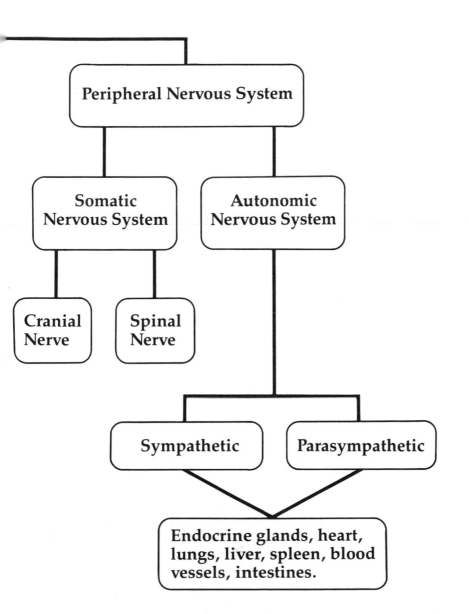

4-1

are stimulated by chemicals (transmitter substances), released in its environment. If enough chemicals are released, then the bag develops holes. A migration of chemicals from inside and outside the neuron takes place, and the neuron loses its negative electric charge as the positively charged chemicals, such as sodium, enter into the holes. The positive charge travels down the axon, and more chemicals are released. The neuron returns to its normal resting state within a few milliseconds. In order for information to travel from one neuron to the next, this process must be repeated. The chemicals just released enter into a space between neurons called the *synaptic cleft* (or *synapse*), neighboring dendrites receive the information, and the message goes forth.

While this seems to be a rather complex process, it is the *only* way that neurons fire off, with the exception that sometimes the whole business may start up spontaneously, and also that the message from some neurons to their neighbors is "don't fire." (These are called inhibitory neurons, whereas the others are referred to as excitatory neurons, for obvious reasons.)

Either a neuron fires off or it doesn't—it has what is called an "all or nothing" property. Strong stimulation, or a lot of chemicals bathing its dendrites, doesn't cause the neuron to fire any differently, only more often. Everything we see, smell, hear—all those images stored up in our memory banks—is based on how many times the neurons fire off, or how many times they don't, and how many and which ones fire at the same time. It's a matter of quantity, not quality. Within this amazing biocomputer called the brain, pathways and structures are consistently linked by the transmission of information by the neurons. There is inevitably cross-talk, so all systems have a modulating influence upon each other.

It is the interrelatedness among neurons and their activities that is critical to the assumption that imagery serves as an integrative mechanism between mental and physical processes. The brain areas associated with image storage, when sufficiently activated by thought (such as occurs when vivid, powerful images are created), can theoretically cause enough neurons to fire repeatedly so the message reverberates through the brain. Thus, imaging a tennis serve activates all those muscles involved. Imaging eating a lemon calls into play glandular secretion, swallowing, grimacing.

In future paragraphs, it is important to keep in mind the way the neurons transmit information. Understanding this, the interconnectedness of the structures will make more sense. There is one hitch, though. The human brain stores and processes much more information than is possible with this mechanism alone. We would literally explode if all the neural circuits were as active as would be required for what is normally in our memory banks. We will discuss more on this problem later.

The Representation of the Image: A Proposed Neuroanatomic Model

The cortex

The cerebral cortex consists of multilayers of nerve cells, distributed and distinguished by the recency with which they appeared in evolutionary development. The cortex is made up of two hemispheres connected by a large fiber bundle called the *corpus callosum*. Cortical areas involved in sensory and motor function of the left side of the body tend to be located on the right side of the cortex, and vice versa. Communication between the two hemispheres is maintained by neurons traversing the corpus collosum, as well as by fibers known as the anterior and posterior commissures, which bridge the thalami.

The right and left hemispheres have developed specialized functions as a consequence of both the evolution of the species and the events of an individual's own developmental history. Knowledge in this area was significantly bolstered by the work of Sperry and Gazzaniga, Bogen and others who studied the results of the "split-brain" surgical procedures.[12] When the fiber bands that connect the hemispheres are severed, seizure activity of severe epilepsy is reduced, but certain kinds of information can no longer travel from one side to the other. In this way, the unique functions of each hemisphere can be known.

Our species apparently had an expanded demand for cortical space to handle the complexities of language, and more and more synapses were recruited into action. Eventually, a sizable portion of the left hemisphere contained the language processing area for approximately 87% of right handers, and 50% of left handers. (Both left handers and those who are ambidextrous may have less lateralized speech function, i.e., both hemispheres contain areas for speech processing.)

The right hemisphere usually contains the specialty components relevant to image storage and retrieval. Here, nonverbal images, rather than words, are used in processing thoughts. The style of information processing also tends to be more nonlinear and less analytic than that of the left hemisphere.[13]

It was not too long ago that the right hemisphere was consistently referred to as the "nondominant" or "minor" hemisphere, because it was assumed to be relatively less involved in human functions. I think it is not less involved at all, but the functions are those less prized when a premium is placed on rational, linear thought and on language. A recent trend, obviously a backlash movement, has been to acclaim the putated functions of the right hemisphere as more special, creative, natural, in touch, in tune, and clearly more desirable than the intellectual mode of the left hemisphere. Considering one side or another of the brain as more vital or more important than the other ignores the fact that the best-functioning people are ambidextrous in their ability to call upon the attributes of both hemispheres. It is true, however, that survival, as well as rehabilitation, is significantly more likely following damage to the left hemisphere than to the right, indicating that life is more dependent upon the functions of the right brain.

Another line of research indicates that while normal individuals have access to both hemispheres, they may prefer to use, or be more adept at using, the mode of one hemisphere over another. Lawyers, for instance, would be expected to use the verbal, left hemisphere; whereas ceramicists, whose work depends upon creating images, would favor the right hemisphere.[14]

The case for the hemispheres

The specific functions that have been attributed to the right hemisphere, and the connections between it and other brain and body components, support the premise that images can and do carry information from the conscious fore to the far reaches of the cells. Consider these findings:

(1) Nonverbal images are a speciality of the right hemisphere. More important to our thesis, *body image* itself is generally lateralized in the right hemisphere. When damage occurs in the parietal lobe of the right hemisphere through a stroke or injury, the patient may fail to recognize part of his or her own body, denying it to the extent that it may not be washed or covered.

(2) The right hemisphere has a predominant role in processing emotional information and in making judgements, and is activated during situations of stress.[15] The importance of the relationship between imagery and emotions was recently demonstrated by Lyman, Bernadin and Thomas, who showed that images were more predominant in situations that were emotionally charged (as compared to situations of neutral or minimal emotion). In discussing

their results, they suggest the role of the image has been underestimated in theories of emotion, and that it may be the determinant for different responses given under similar circumstances.[16]

(3) Because of the implications of the right hemisphere in emotion, it must have a direct relationship with the ANS. This is supported by the existence of a vast network of neural connections between the right hemisphere and the limbic system. The verbal functions of the left hemisphere are one step removed from the autonomic processes, both in evolution and in actual function. Therefore, I submit that *messages have to undergo translation by the right hemisphere into nonverbal, or imagerial, terminology before they can be understood by the involuntary, or autonomic, nervous system.*

(4) Before the imagery that is characteristic of right brain function can be processed into meaningful, logical thought, it must also be accessed and translated by the left hemisphere.[17] *The images so intimately connected with physiology, and with health and disease, are preverbal, or are without a language base,* except what is available from the connections with the left, or speech, hemisphere. If those connections were to be severed and the left hemisphere destroyed or made nonaccessible, untranslated images would continue to affect emotions and alter physiology, but without intellectual interpretation.

A disorder called *alexithymia* (meaning "without words for feelings") is a base in point. Alexithymia has been hypothesized as the basis for what used to be called psychosomatic disorders. It remains a controversial designation, but has a steadily expanding research base.[18] In this condition, it is believed that although emotions and images are experienced, they remain verbally untranslated and are not acted upon in ways that allow them to dissipate. The feelings then seek another outlet, and are diverted into various body systems. The damage caused by this type of expression may eventually be diagnosed as rheumatoid arthritis, ulcerative colitis, asthma, hives, migraine headaches, etc. The etiology of alexithymia is dubious, but functional or structural lesions of the cortical connective pathways, or disruptions between the limbic system and areas of the cortex, as well as deficits in the dopamine striatal tract (the basal ganglia), have been proposed.

(5) The left hemisphere can and does exert deliberate, conscious control over the musculoskeletal system. "Arm extend," "head nod," "put foot down," are all examples of verbal commands that the body hears and can obey quite well, except in the case of pathology or injury. The image system of the right hemisphere can

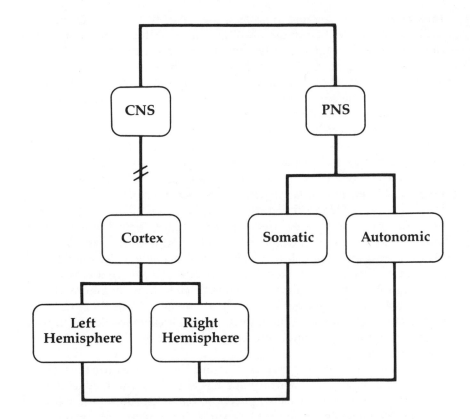

**Autonomic/*Right Hemisphere* = "Unconscious" or Involuntary Functions
Somatic/*Left Hemisphere* = "Conscious" or Voluntary Functions**

4-2

also exert this control by sending thought pictures to the appropriate muscles; for example, by imaging a hand opening like a flower.

The verbal left hemisphere may be conceptualized as an interface with the external milieu, both by virtue of the language exchange between ourselves and others, and the musculoskeletal movements that carry us through space. The imagery of the right side of the brain is the medium of communication between consciousness and the internal environment of our bodies. Both systems are integral to health and well-being. (See Figure 4-2 for a schematic of these ideas.)

A closer look at locale

The right hemisphere covers a lot of territory, so it is prudent to ask just what part of it is the most likely candidate for the image storage place. As we'll note with the discussion on the holographic theory of brain function, images may be redundantly stored in many areas. However, some spots are more likely than others to be the primary stockpile.

The hemispheres are divided into four lobes: the frontal, temporal, parietal, and occipital. Evidence is supportive of some imagery storage in each area, but particularly in the prefrontal or most anterior aspect of the frontal lobes. This area has remained somewhat of a mystery, but tentative research does suggest it is involved in memory storage and emotion, as well. This anterior frontal region is exceedingly well connected to the limbic areas, the part of the brain that processes emotion.[19] The fiber pathways are so numerous, in fact, that the anterior frontal lobes appear as an extension of the emotional system itself—one that has evolved quite recently.

Damage to the anterior frontal lobes results in peculiar deficits. In subhuman primates, lesions in this area produce an impairment of function in tasks requiring a delay in response. On the basis of these experiments, Jacobsen concluded that the anterior aspect of the frontal lobes was necessary for immediate memory, or for use by symbolic memory images.[20] Think what it means to be able to delay a response: Some internal image must be maintained about the response itself and, further, about under what circumstances it is to be emitted. Other studies support the idea that this area is virtually the only part of the brain that is indispensable to the ability to delay responses.

The findings on the role of the anterior frontal lobes are not restricted to monkeys. An outmoded procedure used to treat mental illness involved surgically damaging the frontal lobes, or severing the fiber connections between the frontal lobes and the rest of the brain (frontal lobotomy or lobectomy). The surgical victims were described as not only lacking in emotions, but also unable to fantasize or imagine a future; i.e., they could not hold symbolic images in their heads.[21] Damage to the left frontal lobe tends to produce disruption in verbal tasks, and damage to the right frontal lobe affects image storage and retrieval.[22] It is generally noted that I.Q., as measured by the usual tests, does not suffer as a result of such surgery.

Evidence for involvement of the other right hemispheric lobes in imagery is provided by Humphrey and Zangwill, who described patients with damage to the posterior parietal area of the right hemisphere. They reported little or no dreaming, dim waking imagery, and a lack of ability to function on any tasks requiring visualization: smell, vision, auditory phenomena, and so forth.[23]

A classic disorder called the Charcot-Wibrand syndrome refers to a generalized inability to conjure up visual images.[24] The case described by Charcot involved a man who formerly had a photographic memory. One day, he could no longer recognize faces, including his own; he had no recall of color; and his dreams had lost their visual imagery. His auditory memory was also temporarily disrupted, but his visual memory remained permanently impaired. Critchley claims the locus of such a lesion is the parieto-occipital area, and that the lesion is usually bilateral.

Other evidence suggests such functions may be more lateralized in the right hemisphere. For instance, Milner, DeRenzi, and others have reported on facial memory and memory for meaningless patterns.[25] Both of these are believed to be "pure" visual memory, in that verbal processing is unnecessary for their recall. In both instances, damage to the right temporal lobe disrupts the function. In persons with epilepsy, neural discharge in the right temporal lobe is often associated with dreamlike images or auras that precede seizure activity.[26] Similar observations were made by Wilder Penfield, a surgeon who electrically stimulated areas while patients underwent surgery for epilepsy.[27] Visualizations characteristic of the dreamy state preceding epileptic seizure could be reproduced by stimulation of the right temporal lobe.

The wide dispersion of brain areas involved in imagery, especially visual imagery—indicates the importance of imagery to the survival of the species. Normally, highly important abilities are protected by being redundantly stored, as in this case.

Beyond the cortex
Other areas of the brain besides the cortical hemispheres are obviously necessary to move consciousness downward to contact and alter physiology. The *limbic system,* the outcropping of the image-laden frontal lobes, has already been addressed as a processing area of emotions. The limbic area is a collection of lumps and bumps that constitutes one-third of the brain. Its function in "lower" animals is primarily to react to smells. In mammals, the limbic system has been implicated in feelings of pleasure and reward, pain and punishment, fright, anger, sexual behavior, and the violent acting out of the criminally insane. All of these activities involve the autonomic nervous

system, which, as we will soon note, is critical in tracing the route of the image.

Structurally and functionally, the *hypothalamus* is closely related to neural areas where conscious thought processing occurs and images are formed. The hypothalamus serves in a regulatory capacity over sleeping, eating, body rhythms, temperature, and sexual function; more specifically, it affects heart rate, respiration, blood chemistry, and glandular activity. Of great importance, it has an integral role in regulating the immune system.

Finally, the master gland of the body, the *pituitary*, has both neural and chemical connections to the hypothalamus. It is through these pathways that the hypothalamus manages to alter the hormonal systems of the body, affecting not only the glands, such as the ovaries, testes, adrenals, the thyroid and parathyroid, but also conceivably every organ, tissue and cell.

The evidence for the neuroanatomical bridge between image and cells, mind and body, exists. It is solid, and can be viewed when brain tissue is placed under a microscope. But let us move on to the rest of the story, highlighting the relationship between these visible structures and function.

The Autonomic Nervous System

The *sympathetic nervous system* (SNS) and the *parasympathetic nervous system* (PNS), the two branches of the autonomic nervous system, are both under direct control of the brain. All of the areas mentioned above—the cortex, the limbic system, the hypothalamus and the pituitary—are involved. The target organs are depicted in Fig. 4-3.

The autonomic nervous system pathways between the brain and behavior are usually discussed in terms of the response to stress, although similar pathways, but different chemicals, could be just as readily described for states of sexual arousal, fear and anger, depression, and elation. The point is, the body/mind responds as a unit. No thought, no emotion, is without biochemical, electrochemical activity; and the activity leaves no cell untouched. This follows logically from the facts of how the autonomic nervous system operates. Furthermore, when the chemicals of the target glands are secreted, or even injected, they influence emotional state.

In tracing the pathways from the brain to behavior in a stressful situation, we begin with the perception and conscious recognition that a danger of some sort is present. The danger, of course, need not be "out there," but only fantasized. Vivid mental images of a

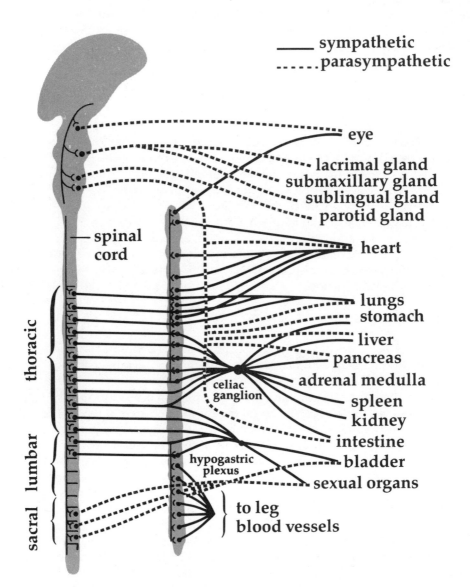

symphathetic
parasympathetic

eye
lacrimal gland
submaxillary gland
sublingual gland
parotid gland

spinal cord

heart

lungs
stomach
liver
pancreas
adrenal medulla
spleen
kidney
intestine
bladder
sexual organs

celiac ganglion

hypogastric plexus

to leg
blood vessels

thoracic

lumbar

sacral

4-3

nuclear attack are completely capable of eliciting a fear response. (On a more pleasant note, fantasizing making love can lead to the same hormonal responses as the "real" thing.) In terms of stress-related disease, it's not the occasional thoughts of unlikely danger that are credited with causing insidious body deterioration, but rather the constant nagging hassles and pressures, the persistent imagery of worrisome events, and cumulative life changes.

A simple model for both emergency stress reactions and chronic stress has been provided by the life work of Hans Selye.[28] In emergency reactions, the sympathetic nervous system predominates, acting in concert with the adrenal glands. The hormones secreted by these glands, adrenalin and noradrenalin, have diffuse mobilization effects on the body. Heart rate increases, sugar is released from the liver for energy, pupils dilate so that vision is enhanced in dim areas, blood clots more rapidly and moves from the peripheral vessels and organs to the muscles and the brain. White blood cell activity increases, preparing the body for emergency repair. The body has primed itself for a war that may never happen, and therefore the state of readiness must dissipate rapidly or else become the enemy within. It is suspected that people with health conditions that involve the cardiovascular system, such as hypertension and migraine headaches, cannot shed the effects of emergency stress quickly. The prolonged reaction may account for the disease itself.

During chronic stress, the mechanisms change. The emphasis is on the secretion of mineralocorticoids and glucocorticoids, the adrenal hormones that are under the influence of the anterior pituitary hormones, including adreno cortico-tropic hormone (ACTH). Again, it is the hypothalamus—which serves as a confluence of conscious function—that influences ACTH release.

When stress is prolonged, the glucocorticoids (hydrocortisone, corticosterone, and cortisone) try to continue the job of maintaining a body fit to fight and repair itself. Nonsugars are transformed into sugar, and blood vessels are sensitized to the adrenal hormones so that action can take place even in the face of fatigue. However, to the great and ultimate detriment of the long-stressed individual, the primary action of ACTH and the glucocorticoids is to reduce inflammatory activity, i.e., the work of the immune system. What was adaptive in the short run can eventually become the cause of every conceivable disease that involves the immune system, including cancer, infection, and autoimmune disorders such as rheumatoid arthritis and multiple sclerosis. The massive changes sustained during prolonged stress go far beyond immune activity to every gland targeted by the pituitary, including those involved in reproduction, growth, and the integrity and well-being of the body at the cellular level.

The network of thoughts/chemicals/behavior is much more sophisticated than was just described, and much more integrated. The intricacies are only beginning to be elaborated. Nobel laureate Julius Axelrod's work suggests the body may cope with different kinds of stressors in different ways, each involving unique neurochemical pathways. His picture is not so bleak as Selye's model of chronic stress and inevitable deterioration. He has evidence suggesting that a body under chronic stress adjusts itself downward, so that fewer of the potentially destructive hormones are released.[29]

Dr. Arthur Samuels, a hematologist and cancer specialist affiliated with UCLA, has recently proposed an elegant theoretical extension of the stress/disease model.[30] He suggests a common group of causes for cancer, heart attack, stroke, and related thrombotic diseases. The causes include chronic stress, a predisposed personality type, and chronic hyperactivation of neural, endocrine, immune, blood clotting (coagulation) and fibrinolytic systems. When stress is prolonged, the clotting mechanism becomes hyperactive, and the fibrinolytic mechanism, which normally inhibits excessive clotting, fails. The resultant blood clots are implicated in both myocardial and cerebral infarctions (heart attack and stroke), as well as other peripheral vascular occlusions. Furthermore, Samuels cites evidence for what he calls "fibrin cocoons," created by blood coagulation, that act as tumor sanctuaries. These cocoons protect the metastasized cancer cells from the T-cells, the body's natural defense against cancer, as well as from chemotherapy and radiation.[31] Under these circumstances, Samuels points out, it is absolutely untenable to expect chemotherapy or radiation to have any effect on metastasized cancer cells, even though these treatments can shrink or debulk the tumor itself.

Whether the Selye model of chronic stress mechanisms is complete or not is a moot issue here. Few would argue with the basic premise that the mind can influence the body in a detrimental way, and that the stressors may well reside in the imagination. The positive pathways that would allow health to follow on the heels of joy and hope are less well-known, and certainly less well accepted. However, we are beginning to have a sense of the chemistry involved, as will be discussed in a subsequent section.

The Holographic Brain

Following Claude Bernard's advice to first analyze the parts and then synthesize the function of the whole, any model of brain function must account for observations that would not be predictable, based solely upon the properties of the isolated neuroanatomic systems. Some of the issues the neuroanatomic model cannot account for in its present conceptualization are these:

(1) Memories don't seem to be stored in any single area, but rather in multiple overlapping areas. And, loss of specific memories is more related to the amount of brain damaged rather than the area damaged.[32]

(2) The abilities initially lost when the brain is damaged by gunshot wounds, tumors, or cardiovascular accident (stroke) often return, even though specific neural regeneration is not believed possible.

(3) Paranormal events that involve receiving, processing, and sending information in ways that do not conform to our understanding of energy transfer are not explainable with the current knowledge of neuroanatomy. This includes the transpersonal healing imagery typically related with shamanic work and with psychic or metaphysical healers.

(4) Phenomena such as phantom limb sensations, persistent phantom pain, and "auras" that extend beyond the corporal self (as seen in Kirlian photographs) call into question the storage of body image, as well as what constitutes physical boundaries of the body.

(5) If only one bit of information is processed per second by the brain, 3×10^{10} nerve impulses per second would be required by the current model of memory storage—an inconceivable amount of neural activity.[33]

(6) The mechanisms of consciousness, or the ability of the brain to consider itself, or thought, or the creation and retrieval of images, elude description in terms of the sheer knowledge of structures and their function as presented in the anatomical models.

At some point, observations from the various levels of science need to be consistent, regardless of whether the data came from a microscope, a telescope, a Rorschach ink blot test, or from sitting around a campfire in Nairobi. The above paradoxes are obvious inconsistencies when compared to the current model of how the brain works. They are facts of human existence, and sooner or later they must be accounted for in terms of brain function and structure.

In order to leap that chasm between the anatomical model of brain function and the nonconforming data, and to encompass the seeming paradoxes, Karl Pribram has proposed that the brain operates like a hologram.[34] Essentially, a hologram is a specially processed photographic record that provides a three-dimensional image when a laser is beamed through it. Its uniqueness lies in the fact that, should it break, any part of the hologram is capable of reconstructing the total image, but with reduced clarity. Like the holograph, the brain also stores information redundantly. Each part of the brain has *some* data on every other part. A shattered piece of the holographic picture can recreate the whole image; the brain areas left intact after damage have the potential for functioning like the missing parts. As we mentioned earlier, memory loss seems to be more a function of *how much* cortex is damaged, and not *where* the damage occurred.

The holographic model, as proposed by Pribram, does not contradict the traditional neuroanatomic description of the brain. Pribram, himself, was a pioneer in creating that model. By no means are all parts of the brain equipotential for every other. The isolated clumps of matter that we call structures, and the nerve pathways, have viable functions that can't be ignored. As Pribram states, "A neural holographic or similar process does not mean, of course, that input information is distributed willy-nilly over the entire depth and surface of the brain."[35] What is challenged by the holographic model, however, is the method of transmitting, storing, and receiving information.

The commonly held and well-tested belief is that the stimulated neuron (nerve cell) carries information down its axon, chemicals are released at the end plates, the chemicals diffuse across the gap or synapse, and then stimulate the activity of neighboring neurons. Pribram claims that information may well be *distributed* this way, but that this is not necessarily the way associations are formed. If associations were to be formed in this manner, the amount of neural transmission defies the imagination—3×10^{10} nerve impulses per second, according to van Heerden's calculations. Pribram's work suggests that we need to reconsider the junction between the neurons, the synaptic cleft, as the area where information is processed, and that the processing may be analogous to the way holograms are formed in photography. "Essentially, the theory reads that the brain at one stage of processing performs its analyses in the frequency domain.

This is accomplished at the junctions between neurons, not within neurons. Thus graded local waxings and wanings of neural potentials (waves) rather than nerve impulses are responsible."[36]

Since there can be as many as a thousand synapses between two neurons, a near infinite number of patterns can be formed. It is speculated that when cortical areas associated with specific types of responses are repeatedly activated, patterns become predictable. Any part of the pattern can regenerate a full-blown perception: a word can trigger the memory of a poem, a smell can recapture a long-forgotten event. Most of the time, our complex behaviors function in this way. We don't think about each separate movement, but rather initiate a rehearsed pattern. In the case of brain damage, the pattern can be recapitulated from remaining data.

Just exactly how the information is encoded and decoded at the neural juncture can be described, as Pribram reasons, in a number of terminologies: statistical, quantal, or mathematical. Pribram prefers to use the holographic analogy of an "instantaneous analogue cross-correlation performed by matched filters."[37] The brain, according to this model, is capable of performing massive numbers of instantaneous computations, based upon the frequencies of data (events) it receives. And, if the holographic photography model is carried still further, the storage has no space/time dimension—the information is everywhere at once.

The holographic model begins to resolve some of the brain/behavior paradoxes, particularly those that relate to the vagaries of memory storage and retrieval. And, if the brain is indeed like a hologram, then it is absolutely unnecessary to have a leg in order for the brain to process "leg" information. It is only necessary to have once had a leg, or even *thought* about having a leg. Either way, storage patterns are set up. There's sensation in the phantom limb, and some control of what the brain perceives as movement.

And what about the paradox of body boundaries: Where do I begin and end? According to the holographic model, we have some choice in the matter. If I decide to wrap my arms around my husband who is fifty miles away, my holographic brain begins to mathematically process what I have experienced about this event: the physical sensations, the emotions, and the symbols I have idiosyncratically adopted—all of which are stored without reference to time or space. The image, if vivid enough, will re-create the whole situation in my being.

The Hologram, the Image, and Health

Pribram says of imagery, "Images and feelings are ghosts—but they are ghosts that inhabit my own and my patients' subjective worlds. They are our constant companions and I want to explain them."[38] He allows that neither behavior nor language function can be adequately explained, despite the press from the behaviorists, without recourse to a map, i.e., an image of some sort. This image can be described with reference to the holographic model of redundant storage at the neural junctures, and the calculation of frequency data.

When images are regarded in the holographic manner, their omnipotent influence on physical function logically follows. The image, the behavior, and the physiological concomitants are a unified aspect of the same phenomenon. The extent to which physical function can be consciously changed would depend upon how much activity is recruited at the neural junctures, and subsequently how many patterns are activated. For this reason, belief systems become critical in matters of achieving health. If you don't believe in the ability to consciously effect physical change with the imagination, you never even try. You don't sort through stored memories, you don't activate patterns, you never give yourself a chance. Healing doesn't happen accidentally, but requires instead either hard mental labor or complete, unbridled faith that what is being done or given to you will create health.

Application of the Holographic Model to Health

According to the principles of the holographic brain, if a person with an illness, say a common cold, wanted to recover in less than seven days, it would be prudent to recruit as many neural patterns of health as possible. Certain systems of mental healing would advise imaging perfect health and harmony. I would suggest imaging the precise body functions involved—throat healing, lungs clearing, the immune system being activated. It might also be important to take Vitamin C (or whatever other medications hold out promise) and imagine it entering into the blood stream, and assisting the immune system. Deep breathing might help, particularly if one imagines the air cleansing stuffy passages. Remembering exactly how it felt to be at the peak of health, and letting the body fall into that mode again, would activate even more neural systems related to health. All of this takes time and the utmost concentration. You may well opt for the natural course of the disease.

On the other hand, it's been my clinical experience that a little practice goes a long way. People don't have much ability to establish healing patterns once they're diagnosed with serious illness. If they don't believe in anything besides modern medicine, when that fails there is nothing else stored in the brain that has been rehearsed sufficiently enough, in the context of health, to effect physical change.

The holographic analogy, together with the processing mode of the neural junctures, has been held to be consistent with several large bodies of work. For example, Akhter Ahsen employs a model quite similar to holography to account for his findings with eidetic imagery therapeutic procedures. The eidetic image is described as a powerful representation that has been impressed on the memory by critical, formative events in the past. The eidetic, by definition, involves physical processes, and part of its massive influence on behavior stems from this association. Ahsen actually considers the eidetic to have a tripartite nature: the image itself (normally conceived as a visual image), a somatic component (a set of body feelings), and a meaning (or cognitive/interpretive) component.[39]

Eidetic therapy involves reviving the eidetics, particularly those believed to have negative consequences on health and well-being. Through a variety of procedures involving sensitive fantasy work, the therapist guides the patient in recovering more adaptive, healthful, imagery. The consequences would, of course, be correlated with change in both somatic and cognitive components, because they comprise a unity. Ahsen and his colleagues attest to the usefulness of this procedure primarily in psychotherapy, but also in dealing with physical disorders believed to have a psychological component.

Biochemistry

In addition to the structures and pathways of the brain and the mathematically based analogy of the holographic mode of information management, biochemistry constitutes still another description of the brain/body interactions. Some of this has been touched upon already in other contexts, and the information included the following facts: Chemicals are involved in the transmission of information from the hypothalamus to the pituitary, in the subsequent release of pituitary hormones, and, in turn, in the production and release of further chemicals from glands such as the adrenals and the ovaries. The chemical path of destruction during chronic stress has been well documented by Selye and investigators following his lead.

Chemicals released at the end points of the axons act to transmit information from one neuron to another, and include serotonin, dopamine, epinephrine, norepinephrine, and acetylcholine. The biochemistry of the brain is now being looked at with the same intensity as that with which tissue and fiber tracts were studied earlier. The preliminary findings offer promise for significant numbers of disorders, as well as new understanding of the role of nutrition in affecting brain function.[40] The relationship between the transmitter chemicals and the imagination is likely to be quite important. Serotonin production and/or inhibition, for example, has been implicated in states of high imagery such as dream sleep, schizophrenia, and the response to lysergic acid diethylamide (LSD).

Feeling states, thoughts, and images can actually *cause* chemicals to be released, and, furthermore, chemicals have the feedback effect of causing feeling states. A chemical balance is integral to the maintenance of health, and that balance can be disrupted or reestablished by all manner of behaviors, including eating, drinking, exercise, and thinking. Blood chemistry and hematology have been noted to be statistically correlated to psychological functioning, and are believed to be significant factors in mental disorders, such as severe depression, anxiety, and manic depression, as well as schizophrenia.[41]

Biochemistry, images, and behavior interact in both the preverbal and the transpersonal methods of healing. Since both types of healing are accomplished in altered states of consciousness, we should examine the biochemical components of these altered states. The methods used to enter the altered state demonstrably provoke dramatic metabolic or biochemical changes. These have been treated in detail in Chapter 1, in the review of the shamanic work. To sum it up briefly here, the changes are occasioned by fasting from food, water, or salt, by sleep and sensory deprivation, temperature extremes, hyper- or hypoventilation, sustained physical activity, and psychoactive substances. Thus, pressing a body to its physiological limits and inducing metabolic shifts are traditional ways to free the constraints on the imagination.

Other methods that induce an altered state of consciousness, such as certain styles of meditation and deep relaxation requiring intense concentration on an object, word, or idea, are also associated with changes in blood chemistry and blood gases.[42] Decreases in oxygen utilization, carbon dioxide production, and blood lactate (a metabolic waste product) have been consistently noted. What Benson has termed the relaxation response is believed to be the opposite in nature of the fight or flight response implicated in so many stress-related disorders, especially cardiovascular disease. In and of itself, relaxation that evokes these physical changes has the potential for reestablishing a physiological homeostasis consonant with health. However, the techniques appear to have efficacy beyond simple relaxation, and are used as preludes to imagery work in both transpersonal and preverbal modes of healing.

Through many complex and varied processes, then, the filters that normally prevent direct mental access to the physical body can be lifted. Most of the ways have in common a means of either removing, or significantly altering, or even competing with, the demands the external environment makes on the brain. The variance in the biochemical outcomes of the different methods described above suggests that the routes to the imagination are many, and the *kind* of biological shift that occurs is relatively less important than whether one occurs at all.

Chemicals of Health

What remains to be examined are the chemicals of health, of joy: the feel-good, get-well chemicals that comprise the drugstore in the mind. What chemicals are associated with happiness? And does happiness, in fact, have something to do with staying well or getting well? What chemicals does the body call forth to heal itself? How can we consciously rally these forces? These are the questions for the medicine of tomorrow. Chapter 6 on immunology will deal, in part, with these issues. But beyond the exciting developments in psychoneuroimmunology, as the new field dealing with behavior and immunology is called, there are other chemical findings that need to be addressed to complete the extant scientific metaphors.

Neuroregulators: Endorphins and Enkephalins

Between 1969 and 1973, two general developments were reported that have extended the appreciation of capabilities of the human body. First, several researchers demonstrated that electrical stimulation of the periaqueductal gray area in the brain produces an analgesia that can be reversed by an analgesia-blocking agent, naloxone. (Naloxone blocks the effect of opiates such as heroin, and is used to counteract drug overdoses.) Second, reports came in of opiate receptors in the central nervous system. Why would the brain have such a specific binding site unless opiates were actually being produced?

And what relationship might the chemicals of the periaqueductal gray area have to other types of opiates? The reasoning led several investigators (chiefly J. Hughes, C. B. Pert, H. L. Li, and their co-workers) to identify, nearly simultaneously, the existence of natural opiates. The terminology used to describe the class of the several compounds includes "endogenous opioid peptides," "endorphins," and "endogenous opioid substances." Various types of endorphins, enkephalins, and lipotropins have been identified within this class. For the most part, they are located in anatomically different areas; however, they are all peptide chains, and tend to have opiate-like properties in addition to their specific functions. Scientists have adopted the convention of referring to the entire family as "endorphins." [43]

The endorphins are found in high concentration in the limbic system, the thalamus, the periaqueductal gray matter, the substantia gelatinosa of the spinal cord—all areas known to be involved in pain transmission. They are also found in areas of the brain that regulate respiration, motor activity, endocrine control and mood. Endorphins are accredited with effecting the increased pain tolerance observed in heroic battle feats, during childbirth, and in significant trauma, although there is little direct evidence for this. It is known that stress increases the concentrations of endorphins in both blood and the brain, with correlated changes in pain tolerance.

The world of pharmacy had great hopes that the endorphins could be synthesized or extracted and prepared for use as a potent, safe narcotic. Unfortunately, they proved to have all the side effects of other pain killers: They create addiction, constipation, confusion, and deficits in learning and memory; they depress respiration, change brain waves, alter motor activity, and produce hormonal imbalances. [44]

The endorphins are affected by things we can do to ourselves and by the imagination. For example, the mechanism of the placebo effect for pain has been demonstrated by Levine and his colleagues to be the endorphins. [45] The placebo effect is a dramatic example of the imagination in action. By sheer dint of the expectation set up following administration of a trusted treatment, pain relief takes place. The method used to demonstrate this was to administer naloxone, morphine, or placebo to fifty-one patients following wisdom tooth extraction. The patients who were given placebos could be classified as placebo responders or nonresponders. For the responders, subsequent administration of naloxone resulted in increased pain levels, indicating that the effects of the natural opiate had been blocked.

It remains to be studied whether the so-called placebo effect in other circumstances, such as in recovery from infectious conditions or serious diseases involving the immune system, can be similarly related to endorphin release. Evidence is mounting, however, that points to their involvement. Relevant to the issue are the studies of Saland et al., who reported that injections of endorphins into the cerebral ventricle of the rat resulted in a macrophage-like cellular response.[46] Investigators from the Research Institute of Scripps Clinic have found that beta-endorphin enhances the ability of T-cells to proliferate;[47] and since beta-endorphin is known to be released from the pituitary during stress, the process of disease may be particularly affected at such times. How it is affected, or in what direction, is not known.

Other evidence suggests the enkephalins are "endogenous immunomodulators"; that is, they assist the immune system in fighting disease. Responses of T-cells taken from cancer patients were enhanced when exposed to enkephalin, according to a report presented by N. P. Plotnikoff at the Second International Conference on Immunopharmacology held in Washington in 1982. Other investigators have reported the presence of opiate receptors on the lymphocytes.[48]

This information on the relationship between endorphins and the immune system, and endorphins and the imagination, puts them in the position of being likely candidates for the healing chemicals of hope. They may well also be the healing chemicals of joy. The whole class of endogenous opiates exhibits anesthetic action, even though their other functions differ. Within the human body, it is impossible to affect the central nervous system centers where pain is processed without also creating some degree of euphoria. This is precisely the problem with chronic use of major pain killers: Almost everyone likes to be euphoric, and addiction is possible within a matter of weeks. If being happy is healing, and laughter is medicine, then the biochemical mechanism is no doubt some aspect of the endorphin complex.

Activities that are reputed to induce a natural high, such as running or other aerobic exercise, have been associated with increased blood levels of endorphins. The more intense the exercise, and the more it's repeated, the greater the endorphin secretions.[49]

Goldstein offers the first objective evidence that music, too, can create changes associated with the endorphins. He investigated what he called "thrills," characterized by tingling sensations, which accompany emotionally arousing stimuli. Approximately one-half of the 249 subjects questioned reported that they experienced such thrills in response to music. In some of his subjects, the sensation was attenuated with naloxone. Music, as pointed out in Chapters 1 and 2, has always had a role in traditional healing ceremonies. Furthermore, it has been used as "audio analgesia," especially by dentists, for some time. Also, music therapy is recognized as a legitimate area of study in many universities. Usually music is considered to benefit the patient primarily because it serves as a distraction from the aversive situations of illness or treatment. Goldstein's work suggests the therapeutic aspects of music may be biochemical as well, and calls for extensive study into this issue.[50]

And, if you've ever drowned your sorrows in a hot fudge sundae, you have a distinctly personal knowledge of how sweetness can assuage misery. Sweetness does indeed plug into a pleasure center. Now, there is a tentative report supporting what we suspected all along. Sweet tastes are associated with endorphin release *and* with increased pain tolerance.[51] This information may resolve some puzzles: why you can train a rat to do just about anything with a chocolate chip cookie or even a watery saccharin solution as a reward; why chronic pain patients eat sweets, often to the exclusion of anything else; and why low-income children have so much money in their pockets to buy candy on the way home from school. Fifty cents a day buys the cheapest, quickest joy the poor can afford.

Other self-healing chemicals include alpha-melanocyte-stimulating hormone, a recently identified brain peptide which can fight fever 25,000 times more effectively, molecule for molecule, than aspirin. It is hoped that this ongoing work, conducted by James Lipton, Mark Murphy and Dave Richards at the University of Texas Health Science Center in Dallas, will eventually provide an alternative for the fever drugs that are on the market. I would suggest that these internal fever-fighters, too, are likely to be more effective when brought under conscious control than when used as pills.

Another natural healer is histamine, a chemical released to aid the immune system in its attack. Blushing, itching, the chest and face flush of sexual arousal, hives, and allergies are all histamine overreactions, all intimately associated with emotions—and, hence, on theoretical bases, amenable to conscious direction. I feel certain that the results we have obtained with temperature biofeedback on individuals who have had delayed wound healing are in part a result of their ability to control histamine release, and thereby speed the healing response. (Increased temperature is normally thought to reflect increased blood flow; however, a histamine reaction would also elevate skin temperature slightly because of the signal it gives to the vessels to dilate.) This remains to be tested, as does the entire natural pharmacopeia, in terms of the limits of its direction by the imagery process.

Behavioral and Social Science: Imagination as Psychotherapy

5

. . . the rise of civilization in the last 2000 years reads like a history
of the social suppression of visualization and therefore a denial of
one of our most basic mental processes. For visualization *is* the way
we think. Before words, images were.

Don Gerrard, 1975
Introduction to Samuels and Samuels' Seeing with the Mind's Eye

Having reviewed the evidence of the physical sciences, let us turn
to the behavioral and social sciences and see what implications the
research in these fields has on the role of imagination in healing.
Behavioral science and social science, as the terms will be used in
this chapter, will include the observations of those scientists who
study the behavior of the individual or consider the cultural milieu in
relation to the imagination and healing. They are professionals who
might well regard the functions and structure of subatomic particles,
tissues, and organs as related to behavior, but *most* (not all, certainly) do not include these levels within their analyses. For this
reason, the material is a departure from the basic thesis of this book,
which treats the image as intimately connected to physiology, and
attempts to demonstrate the correlation with data from the basic
sciences. However, although the position of the behavioral and social scientists may be incomplete, it is not invalid; and it effectively

complements other levels of science in terms of helping us understand how the image interacts with behavior and ultimately with health.

Image as Hypothetical Construct

In the behavioral and social sciences, "image" is treated as an hypothetical construct, an intervening variable between the stimulus/input and the response/output. As such, the image finds itself in the quite respectable company of the other great issues studied: learning, motivation, memory, and perception. None of these concepts is regarded as unreal, or unworthy of study, or beyond change, even if they are invisible. Even though one can't observe "learning" or "motivation," but only note changes in behavior as a predictable consequence of some stimulus, laws have been developed to describe how these factors operate.

The most reductionistic level of all science, quantum physics, ultimately studies only the hypothetical construct. Subatomic particles have not been observed directly, any more than has the image. The form and function of both can only be implied by introducing an input variable and measuring an output variable; hence, the term *intervening variable*. Both behaviorism and quantum physics are measuring ghosts, with commendable precision, by quantifying the antecedent and consequent events. The status of these ghosts as hypothetical constructs might well be only temporary, pending the development of a technology that would allow for more direct observation of the phenomena itself. On the other hand, if, as the quantum physicists suggest, the imagination is the basis for all form, all matter, the ghosts may remain.

The position of the social and behavioral sciences, restated, is that the image is a putated event that is influenced by both the internal and external environment, or in a relationship between stimulus and response. In this schema it is not necessary to describe the image in a phenomenological sense. That would be less parsimonious (i.e., would require more explanatory variables) and may not add to either predictability or controllability. Nor do most behaviorists find it necessary to engage in "physiologizing" or speculating on the neuroanatomic and biochemical correlates of the image.

In the behavioral sciences, the image, as an intervening variable or hypothetical construct, can be used as a tool for restructuring the meaning of a situation, so that it no longer has the power to create distress. Implicit in this interpretation is a concomitant reduction of anxiety or other negative emotional consequences, and also a reduction in behaviors that might be considered responses to the anxiety-provoking situations. In this light, imagery could be viewed as an important instrument for preventing the disorders that are known to be either induced or exacerbated by stress. To date, virtually every disease under scrutiny has been associated with stress in some measure, including cardiovascular disease, arthritis, cancer, diabetes, the autoimmune disorders, ad infinitum.

In addition to blaming the unremitting stress-responses, the prevailing notion is that other behaviors, such as improper habits of nutrition, sleep, sanitation, exercise, smoking, and excessive intake of toxic substances, actually cause or provoke much of what is considered physical disease. Demonstrating imagery as an instrument of behavioral change further substantiates its position as an intervention device. The imagination as healer is therefore identified and justified by the social and behavioral paradigm without recourse to either reductionistic levels of science, or to supernatural, transpersonal explanations.

Treating Illness versus Treating Disease

Several new issues are raised when the behavioral or cultural perspective is brought into the scientific metaphor, issues that were not a cause for concern as long as healing was discussed on the cellular or even the subatomic level. Specifically, what is healing, anyway? As Arthur Kleinman points out, *healing* is an embarrassing word that exposes the archaic roots of medicine, long buried under the facade of modern health care.[1] Studies of cross-cultural healing are doomed to fail precisely because of the problem with, and reluctance in, defining healing in different traditions. Even with a cosmopolitan medical system, there is no agreement on what constitutes healing. Patients and physicians maintain two separate sets of criteria with which they judge medical outcome, with physicians tending to identify biological change, and patients opting for the more subjective components of "feeling better," as the appropriate variables.[2]

Kleinman goes on to describe two radically different healing functions that are typical of contemporary and traditional forms of health care: controlling the sickness, and providing meaning for the individual's experience of it.[3] He then offers separate definitions of disease and illness: "Let us call disease any primary malfunctioning in biological and psychological processes. And let us call illness the secondary psychosocial and cultural responses to disease, e.g., how the patient, his family, and social network react to his disease."[4] This distinction between illness and disease, the attempts to treat one or the other, and the culturally appropriate definition of healing are, in my opinion, the most vital and overlooked aspects of modern medical care.

Those systems that use the imagination in its fullest preverbal and transpersonal sense, then, would not only be influencing the biological or psychological processes, but also treating the illness. A Mohawk elder, Ernie Benedict, made the observation in another way: "The difference that exists is that the White doctor's medicines tend to be very mechanical. The person is repaired but he is not better than he was before. It is possible in the Indian way to be a better person after going through a sickness followed by the proper medicine."[5]

The material of the behavioral and social scientists is largely concerned with illness and not disease, with the subjective (or psychological) factors, and with behavioral change. For those who do field work, this is practically mandated, often by their own limited training in measuring the disease variables. Also, it is behavior and verbal reports, not blood or x-rays, that are available for analysis in the field settings.

Territory of the Behavioral and Social Sciences in Health

As I move through this information, I will continue to wrestle with both the semantic and cognitive problems of discussing health. Based upon the data from physiology, biochemistry, and quantum physics, there can be no clear distinction between mental and physical disease, or a difference in territory of the medical and social/behavioral sciences. Mental/physical, body/mind, are false dichotomies, peculiar to our culture. Schizophrenics have biochemical abnormalities; does that make schizophrenia a physical or mental disorder? Cancer, diabetes, and heart disease have predictable psychological correlates. What category, then, must they be in? The dichotomy becomes even more detrimental as intervention proceeds along territorial lines of the various specialities.

The imagination is frequently described in the behavioral literature as most efficacious in healing imaginary diseases—using thought forms to fight thought forms. Imagination is also commonly considered part of a coping mechanism in the configuration of the illness, the response to the disease. It is not surprising that the behavioral work in imagery focuses primarily on mental disorders. An exception to this is those diseases that have physical symptoms, but are believed to have psychological origins, i.e., the so-called psychosomatic diseases (asthma, migraine, ulcerative colitis, hives, rheumatoid arthritis, essential hypertension, etc.).

The term *psychosomatic* has produced an unfortunate cul-de-sac in thinking, even among the learned. Designating something "psychosomatic" indicates that both the psyche and the soma are involved in a delicate interplay. Lipowski defines the scope of psychosomatic medicine as (1) a scientific discipline concerned with the *relationships* of biological, psychological, and social determinants of health and disease; and (2) a set of postulates that embody a holistic approach to medicine.[6] Yet, the term has come to imply that the psychological problem was primary, leaving an erroneous impression of physical disorders that are "all in the head," or worse, "an improbable hybrid of clinical thinking, physiological speculation and psychoanalytic theory."[7] Some authors, including Pelletier,[8] claim that as much as ninety percent of all disease has psychological components; therefore, either the psychosomatic concept needs to be correctly defined in the medical and psychological literature, or a new designation given (such as "psychophysiological"), where it is understood that mental and physical phenomena are interactive.

"Conversion hysteria" is another category of interest, and one frequently chosen to describe the etiology of the conditions of those who undergo rapid physical betterment through the use of the imagination. The classical hysteric is one who, being unable to face psychic conflict, subconsciously diverts the conflict into the body. Upon examination, the symptoms have no organic basis. The patient is believed to benefit because a convenient escape from an unsolvable situation is provided by adopting the sick role. Blindness, loss of speech or hearing, and partial or complete paralysis are typical symptoms.

So, the territory of the behavioral and social sciences should include all disorders, all deviations from adequate or adaptive functioning, but is normally restricted in viewpoint to the traditional categories of mental disease and coping strategies for physical disease. Neurosis, psychosis, depression, anxiety, and schizophrenia are all frequently mentioned in the context of imaginal healing.

Formats for Study

There are several ways the behavioral and social scientists have studied the imagination. One is to consider the image and its role in cognition and behavioral change. Another method is to observe and interpret the behavior of individuals in systems that use the imagination in a healing format. The latter topic tends to involve field work, with the analyses made by sociologists, anthropologists, psychologists, and psychiatrists interested in cross-cultural healing, while the former is normally conducted in a research laboratory or clinical setting.

Other approaches, which are growing in application and influence, are conducted by those behaviorists and social scientists who do clinical work and research in the area of physical disease, and who are appreciative of the mind and body interactions. They are reluctant to segment out what belongs to the "mental" and what to the "physical," both in etiology and in intervention, but most of them work within and grant allegiance to the medical model. They are as likely to be found plying their trade in cardiac rehabilitation units, cancer treatment centers, and pain control programs, as in health research settings. While the majority are research rather than clinically oriented, the clinical tools that are employed include counseling and psychotherapy, cognitive strategies for coping, behavior modification, biofeedback, hypnosis, patient education, meditation and relaxation techniques, and imagery. Their research interests range broadly through topics of health behaviors, psychological etiology and correlates of disease, prevention and intervention strategies, and epidemiology. The professional affiliation of such individuals has come to be known as "behavioral medicine" or "health psychology," or in some sectors as "humanistic medicine."

Holistic medicine has been deliberately omitted from the behavioral and social categories for several reasons. First, because it is an amorphous designation that has generously embraced healers and healing methods of every conceivable type, it is impossible to describe such diversity. Second, while most who consider themselves holistic medicine practitioners are open to healing with the imagination (indeed, are highly supportive), their interest has been in clinical applications rather than in the establishment of an empirical foundation. With the exception of the American Holistic Medical Association and Holistic Nursing Associations, most groups do not have either an academic or professional affiliation. Regardless of the efficacy or soundness of its interventions, holistic medicine has not yet made a distinctive contribution to the scientific efforts in this area.

Growing Interest in the Image

The research-oriented behavioral scientists have done much to analyze the image using the methods of science. During the last two decades, they've employed sophisticated statistical tools and astute clinical perceptions to bring the imagination out of the ranks of ostrasized topics, into the arena of acceptability. Research articles and reviews of the literature in journals and books have proliferated at an amazing rate. The maturity of approach and interest in the subject are evidenced by the factions that have formed, supporting one or another theoretical framework. Three active national associations include a diversity of members with the singular interest of the imagination. The *Journal of Mental Imagery* was founded in 1977 as a professional multidisciplinary forum, to include articles on the experimental, clinical, and theoretical aspects of imagery.

Professional groups that have either a research or clinical interest in the field include psychologists as a majority, but also physicians (particularly psychiatrists), art and music therapists, educational specialists, theologians, and anthropologists. Within psychology, the image has been researched from the perspective of clinical work and psychopathology, memory and learning, perception and sensory psychology. Several excellent edited works have been published recently that attempt an overview of literally thousands of articles and opinions on this topic.[9] The appropriateness and value of the image as a suitable study for the behavioral sciences is clearly established.

In surveying this monumental amount of work, the greatest disappointment is that so little can be abstracted as directly relevant to a scientific metaphor for the imagination as healer. On the other hand, when the definition of health includes mental health in all its complexity, adaptation to cultural mores, learning to one's capacity, an expanded appreciation of the arts, and the development of creativity, then it is all relevant.

Imagery in the Clinical Setting

The use of imagery in the psychotherapeutic setting has a vast, rich history, as well as existing still in the contemporary fore. The work has been thoroughly reviewed by Anees Sheikh and Charles Jordan, who cite 225 references, ranging from the early work of Freud, Jung, and the European schools to the approaches of the modern therapists.[10] This scholarly article deserves to be read in its entirety. The following table contains only a partial listing of the methods and persons involved in imagery therapy, and is included primarily to demonstrate the breadth of application.

The conditions that are reported as having been successfully treated with imagery by the behaviorists are those believed to have origins in behavior or cognitive problems. Included are phobias and anxieties (fears of snakes, the opposite sex, heights, open places, public speaking, injections); depression; conditions related to habits such as obesity, smoking, alcohol and drug abuse; insomnia; impotency; and "psychosomatic symptoms."

As Sheikh and Jordan point out, though, clinicians are more interested in describing applications of imagery than in doing solid experimental work to validate "the pivotal process assumptions that underlie these procedures."[11] On the other hand, the behavioral therapists have done a great deal of research, but neglected to formulate a theoretical base. Additionally, they have tended to place the image outside the individual, assuming it operated on covert behavior as other principles were known to operate on overt behavior.[12] What is necessary is a testable model which can either demonstrate the validity of the behaviorists' assumptions, or else define the role of the image on behavior in some other way. Offerings in that vein appear below.

How Imagery Changes Behavior

Donald Meichenbaum has developed several techniques that use the imagination as a clinical tool, including "coping imagery" and "stress innoculation." Accordingly, he has formulated a three-process model that accounts for and develops the effect of cognitive factors (such as the image) as mediators of behavioral change. The first phase of his training involves developing self-awareness of both behaviors and internal events such as thoughts, feelings, and physiological reactions. Secondly, new, adaptive thoughts (images) are introduced to replace the distressing, maladaptive ones. And finally, the person is encouraged to generalize the newly learned thoughts and behaviors outside of the clinic, in real-life situations. The basic treatment model is believed to involve cognitive restructuring, and is quite popular among behaviorists.[13]

Meichenbaum, in describing the effect of his and other imagery-based therapies, feels the underlying mechanisms are (1) a feeling of control which is gained as a function of rehearsing the images; (2) the changed internal dialogue that becomes associated with the maladaptive behaviors; and (3) the mental rehearsal of the adaptive responses.[14]

Jerome Singer proposes that the efficacy of imagery lies in (1) the ability of the person to discriminate fantasy processes; (2) clues from the therapist on ways to approach uncomfortable situations; (3) the rehearsal of alternatives; and (4) consequent decreases in fear in approaching situations that were previously avoided.[15] Generally, the person gains a sense of mastery through the imagery process.

Frequently, imagery strategies are used to combat pain associated with a variety of conditions, especially headache, low back pain, and dental pain. The patient is advised to relax and image pleasant scenes, which are either guided by the therapist or created through the patient's individual fantasies. An often proposed mechanism is that imagery serves as a distraction, and pain tolerance is thereby increased.[16] Others propose that imagery is most effective in pain control, particularly when it is pleasant,[17] and when it promotes attributions of self-control.[18]

Healing with the Imagination as a Cultural Phenomena

We turn, now, to another area where healing with the imagination is described in the language of behavior and in the context of social systems: the broad area of nonmedical, cultural or folk healing practices. Ethnopsychiatrists have been especially prolific in delineating the reasons why the practices work, and often draw parallels between the techniques of the native healer and their own. Naturally, their focus is on the mental aspects of disease, and like the other behaviorists, they regard imagery as best suited for the imaginary (nonphysical) diseases, or as a coping mechanism. The "timeworn and unproven psychoanalytic theories which . . . have introduced so much obscurantism into this subject . . ."[19] will be assiduously avoided in the following discussion.

The methods of study in this area are normally based upon observation, with actual experimentation being unfeasible and somewhat irrelevant. For this kind of material, careful, objective reporting, particularly if it is accompanied by some quantification, is gen-

Imagery and Psychotherapy

School/Technique	Author/Date
Autogenics	Schultz & Luthe (1959)
Auto Hypnosis	Vogt (Jordan 1979)
"	Frank (1910)
Behavioral	Anderson (1980)
Cognitive Restructuring	Meichenbaum (1977, 1978)
Conditioned Reflex Therapy	Salter (1949)
Convert Conditioning Techniques	Cautela (1977)
Death Imagery	Achterberg & Lawlis (1981)
"	Sheikh (1979)
Dialogue Method	Kretschmer (1969)
"	Happich (1932)
"	Binet (1922)
"	Caslaut (1921)
Directed Reverie	A. Freud (Compton 1974)
"	Silberer (Kosbab 1974)
Directed Reverie	Guillery (1945)
"	Clark (1925)
Eidetic Psychotherapy	Ahsen (1965)
Emergent Uncovering	Reyher (1977)
"	Horowitz (1968, 1970, 1978)
Emotive-Reconstructive Therapy	Morrison (1980)
Focusing	Gendlin (1978)
Gestalt (humanistic/transpersonal)	Perls (1979)
Group Psychotherapy	Saretsky (1977)
Guided Affective Imagery	Leuner (1977, 1978)
Guided Imaging	Wolpin (1969)
Imagery/Diagnosis	Yanovski & Fogel (1978)
Imagery/Hypnosis	Sheehan (1979)
Imagery Substitution	Janet (1898)
Implosion/Flooding	Rachman (1968)
"	Stampfl & Lewis (1967)
Inner Advisor Technique	Jaffee & Bresler (1980)
Intensive Journal	Progoff (1963, 1970)
Oneirodrama	Fretigny & Virel (1968)
"	Desoille (1965)
Psychoanalytic	Freud (Singer & Pope, 1978)
"	Jung (1960)
"	Kanzer (1958)
"	Goldberger (1957)
"	Kepecs (1954)
"	Jellinek (1949)
Psycho-Imagination Therapy	Schorr (1972, 1978)
Psycho-Synthesis	Assagioli (1965)
Rational Emotive Therapy	Ellis (1981)
"	Lazarus, Abramovitz (1962)
Reconditioning	Williams (1923)
Systematic Desensitization	Wolpe (1958, 1969)

physical disorders; general tool of psychotherapy to promote free
association
recuperative influence and enhanced general efficiency
deep relaxation and hypnogogic
review theoretical and applications
cognitive process to change behavior; stress innoculation; coping strategies
behavioral treatment phobias
operant and social learning procedures
imagery in dying patients
accepting death
meditative techniques in psychotherapy
therapeutic approach using predetermined scenes
to reveal unconscious subpersonalities; "provoked introspection"
psychic development; extrasensory experience
free and directed imagery with children
symbolic nature of images
directed reverie and neuromuscular change
access to childhood memories, narcissistic neurosis
image, somatic pattern, and meaning (ISM)
free association of images
imagery in cognitive psychology
elicitation and integration of feelings
recognition of feelings, general psychology and physical problems
fantasy and psychodrama
imagery methods with group
systematic guided imagery
behavioral treatment; avoidance behavior
visual imagery projection of Rorschach
literature review
overcoming hysteria, idea substitution
extinction of fear response
           ''
use of "inner advisor" for diagnosis, therapy
inner dialogue for self awareness, change
directed day dreams
           ''
physical disorders and general tool of psychotherapy to promote free
association
"active imagination" in psychotherapy
images used for uncovering purposes and to follow motivation state
images used in clarifying relationships between somatic sensations and life
events
images as way of overcoming blocks in free association
imagery as a way of approaching unconscious "on its own terms"
existential and phenomenological approach
eclectic and humanistic, symbolic emphasis
work through irrational fears
behavioral treatment with children's phobias
behavioral treatment
behavioral disorders; phobias; counterconditioning

erally agreed upon as an acceptable data base. Other scientists, such as Jerome Frank, rely on the anthropological reports for data, and speculate and draw conclusions from their own fields of expertise.

For the purposes of this particular topic, I will classify the shamans, the curanderos, the so-called witchdoctors, the medicine men and women, the indigenous practitioners, as well as contemporary religious or faith healers, as folk healers. Within any given cultural setting, though, the titles may designate different skill levels. Especially, the shaman is singled out historically as having the greatest expertise in working with the imagination. In making the observations on the healing mechanism, the behavioral and social scientists usually do not recognize the distinction among the healers, and their remarks are reasonably applicable to anyone who uses healing rituals that are not regarded as having active medicinal properties.

The Principle of Rumpelstiltskin: Diagnosis

In common with the contemporary physician, the nonmedical healer is granted the privilege of diagnosis. E. Fuller Torrey expounds upon the importance of this task, calling it the "principle of Rumpelstiltskin," after the old fairy tale where magic appeared when the correct word was spoken. According to Torrey, the very act of naming is therapeutic, conveying the reassurance that someone actually understands. The typical belief is that if the problem can be understood, *or even named*, it can be cured. The patient feels relief, and can face the outcome in a state of calmness. Only those who hold positions of great respect in any culture can effectively do the naming. They must hold a world view in common with the patient, and the diagnosis must be relevant to that world view in order to be effective. (As Torrey says, this poses a significant problem in any cross-cultural attempt at psychotherapy; one would presume that applies to any attempt at cross-cultural medicine, as well.)[20]

The principle of Rumpelstiltskin is vital in any health setting. Patients look far and wide for a diagnosis they can accept, regardless of whether it matters a whit as far as treatment is concerned.

Purveyors of Hope, Self-Esteem and Cultural Reintegration

The most prevalent themes throughout the literature, and the most relevant to the metaphor under consideration, are that the folk healer is successful because of an ability to engender hope, to bolster faltering self-esteem, and to assist the disfunctional individual in finding a comfortable acceptance within the community. These very qualities are pointed to as significant deficits in the cosmopolitan medical practices, and as reasons for emulating more of the behaviors of the folk healer. There is also an assumption that such efforts will lead to feelings of well-being, if not to actual changes in the corporeal body; i.e., they will improve the illness, if not the disease. Other writers describe the potential for positive change in both disease and illness.[21]

Drs. Ness and Wintrob claim that the effectiveness of folk healers rests in their ability to capitalize on the patients' feelings of dependency, diminished self-esteem and anxiety, to intervene with promises of recovery. The therapeutic ritual provides a plan for the entire community to follow, and a sense of mastery and purpose is lent to all who participate. The patients' self-esteem is improved by being the focal point for the activity. And, according to these writers, when the healer calls upon supernatural forces, the patient receives further validation of being worthy of the ultimate form of help.[22]

Weatherhead characterizes the underpinnings of healing by faith (and, hence, the imagination) as a condition of "expectant trust."[23] The folk healers have the capacity to elicit such trust if they present themselves as charismatic figures or if their reputation for having special gifts has become known to the patient. When hope returns, the patients feel less depressed, stronger, and more energetic—factors believed to be associated with accelerated healing,[24] or at least an improvement in the illness.

Torrey cites several characteristic factors that serve to engender trust in healers of all types: the trip or pilgrimage to visit the healer (distance seems to be important here); the impressiveness of the building or edifice and the contents therein; the distinctiveness of the healer's demeanor; his or her training credentials; and a pervasive air of power and mystery, even fear.[25] The esteem of the patient is increased by merely being in the presence of and receiving the undivided attention of such an impressive, important person. The fears and anxieties of the relatives, which may help sustain the sick role of the patient, are also abated with the knowledge of impending help.[26]

A description of the shaman is appropriate here: "He is readily distinguishable from the laity by his taciturnity, his grave and solemn countenance, his dignified step, and his circumspection. All of these peculiarities tend to heighten his influence, and, by rendering his appearance impressive and suggestive of superiority, serve to increase his control over the people."[27]

The wide and nearly-classic literature on helplessness can be invoked here, following the solid experimentation of Martin Seligman and his colleagues, as well as the earlier reports of Cannon on voodoo death.[28] Helplessness can literally be lethal, or barring that, significantly detrimental to the individuals' health and well-being. Distinctive behavioral changes have been noted in several species when they were confronted with a situation over which they had no control. The changes could be anthropomorphically described as "giving up," and are accompanied by evidence of physical deterioration. Helplessness in humans is normally associated with severe depression, apathy, and loss of energy, even before the clinical manifestation of disease. The gist of the work that is relevant to the folk healers is that when control or hope is reinstated, it is accompanied by physical and behavioral improvement. The purveyors of hope, in this context, are offering a healing commodity.

Transpersonal/Spiritual Healing

The behavioral and social scientists usually ignore the transpersonal or spiritual component of folk healing altogether. Occasionally, the associated rituals will be described as factors in improving the psychological outlook of the patient. Jerome Frank's remarks are typical in this regard, and most resources surveyed either quote him or offer a permutation of the same thought, viz: The "methods of primitive healing involve an interplay between patient/healer, group, and the world of the supernatural; this serves to raise the patient's expectancy of cure, help him to harmonize his inner conflicts, reintegrate him with his group and the spirit world, supply a conceptual framework to aid this, and stir him emotionally."[29] He goes on to say that the function of the total process is to combat demoralization and to strengthen the patient's sense of self-worth.

The spiritual, transpersonal aspect of the imaginary work is viewed somewhat differently by Guenter Risse, specialist in the history of medicine. He believes the "elaborate network" of spiritual relationships that are created by the society in which such healing takes place are a built-in escape hatch, which allows humans to transcend "an apparent determinism imposed by the supranatural components of the cosmos." He mentions that even today people are attracted to the occult to transcend the bonds of scientific determinism. The rituals, divination procedures, and the therapeutic actions are derived, he believes, from a magico-religious world view. "They appeal to the emotional irrational components of the psyche, providing satisfaction for our metaphysical needs and products of the imagination."[30]

The religious beliefs can also be addressed as an aspect of learning theory. That is, they are classified as superstitious behaviors, and defined as instances that may have been powerfully reinforced by coincidental events in the near or distant past of the tribe. The appearance of an intermittant reinforcer has a known and intensive ability to sustain human behavior (prime examples are slot machines). According to these principles, healing events that were in fact "spontaneous remissions" or instances of self-limited disorders, may have "accidentally" been associated with the supernatural petitions and magico-religious activities of the healers. Superstitious behaviors also have the effect of reducing anxiety and generating hope during the interim between illness and recovery. In experimental situations, superstitious behaviors have been described as bridging the time span between stimulus and reinforcement, or as a chain of behaviors to mediate delays between events.[31]

The Rituals

The essence of folk healing lies in the ritual and not in what is normally conceived of as medicine. Therefore, the social and behavioral observers have attempted to describe and/or explain any healing effects in terms of what the rituals might mean, were they to be conducted in more modern circumstances.

The consensus is that the value of the ritual lies in the following: (1) The lengthy preparations usually required before the healing ritual provide something for the relatives to do to show concern; (2) ritual preparations and participation are a way for both the patient and the community to feel in control of what appeared to be a hopeless situation; (3) relationships within the community are cemented and group solidarity is enhanced; (4) the drama and esthetics of the ritual are soothing and distracting; (5) the features of the ritual cement the ties between patient and a group from which he or she may have felt alienation; (6) the patient can sense relief through believing that harmony between himself/herself and the spirit world is established; (7) the rituals and symbols serve to interpret the meaning of disease, as well as the patient's role, in a cultural context; (8) the patient is stirred emotionally by the intensity of the ritual, and this further increases hope or expectant trust that something important will happen; (9) the cost of healing rituals is considerable in most cultures (including Western medicine, needless

to say), and may entail the preparation of more prized and nutritious foodstuffs, again enhancing the self-esteem, hope and pride
of the patient; (10) when psychoactive preparations are used, or
when altered or dissociative states are entered into as a consequence
of the ritual, the power of the healer is validated by such unusual
experiences and these reinforce the spiritual belief system.

Ness and Wintrob provide interesting observations on the reason the dissociative states entered into by both healer and healee
might be effective. They assert that the experience makes the patient
more susceptible to suggestions made by the healer, and that the
dissociative state may be cathartic, if the patient is given permission to behave in ways that would be socially unacceptable in other
contexts.[32]

The psychotherapeutic value of the ritual has been well expressed by Wolfgang Jilek, a psychiatrist and anthropologist who
has conducted field work in East Africa, Haiti, South America,
Thailand, Papua New Guinea, and among the Indians in Western
Canada. While the remarks below were observations made on the
spirit dancing of the Coast Salish Indians, they are applicable to
almost any healing ritual. Jilek has identified components of *activity*
or *occupational therapy*, and noted that *group therapy* is relevant, with
group solidarity and cohesion frequently expressed. The ritual provides the opportunity for *cathartic abreaction*, which is believed to
liberate one from pent-up emotional tensions as situations are re-
lived. *Psychodrama* or dramatic acting is a conspicuous feature of
many healing rituals. In the modern therapy setting, psychodrama
has the purpose of allowing the person to express issues or act out
in a controlled, supportive setting. And finally, he notes the psycho-
hygienic effect of intense *physical activity*. Indeed, recent research, as
well as ancient tradition, suggest physical activity can combat depression, as well as enhancing physical fitness. Ritual work may
involve chanting, dancing, and singing for days, or, in the case of
the spirit dancers, it lasts for months.[33]

Further points are made by Robert Bergman, a psychiatrist who
studied in a Navaho "School for Medicine Men," and who practiced
psychiatry among the Navaho for several years. He notes that during
the lengthy Navaho ceremonies or "sings," the prolonged and intense nature of the contact makes it inevitable that conflicts be revealed, which, if skillfully handled, can then be resolved. He also
sees the rituals as a time of moratorium and turning point.[34]

The theme that weaves through all the behavioral and social

scientists' work on illness is that much of illness is caused by disharmony—disharmony with nature, with self, and especially with the
community. When the entire community becomes a healing network, when time is devoted to focusing acutely on the problem,
and when the patient's support system becomes active and obvious,
healing of many ailments becomes possible.

6 Immune Odyssey: Mind and Disease

I have little patience with scientists who take a board of wood, look for its thinnest part, and drill a great number of holes where drilling is easy.

Albert Einstein

The final chapter of this book is about mind: the link between disease and the environment, the controlling force of the body's protection system, the storehouse for the secrets of health and disease. The study of these factors is the subject matter of one of the most exciting fields in science today, *psychoneuroimmunology*. This is the area in which the research on the role of the imagination in health has been most clearly delineated using scientific method.

The mysteries of the crippler and killer diseases will be solved, not by finer and finer microscopic inspection of diseased tissues, but by careful study of the very unusual people who either defy the odds by recovering or who evidence unusual immunity and don't become ill in the first place. While causes for cancer, arthritis, diabetes, multiple sclerosis—all the incurables—elude medical science, a great deal is known about the behavior of these diseased cells and tissues and organs. This field, pathophysiology, has reaped the benefits of the age of high technology. Lasers, computers, and telemetry have become part of medicine's searchlight, illuminating the failings of the human body. Armed with their gleaming probes, scientists have riveted their attention on the description of the disease process as an isolated phenomenon, nearly separate from the host that bears it. This has proven to be an inordinately fruitful investigative style, yielding information unparalleled in history. But it has come to a point of diminishing returns. Billions of dollars are spent on this and that war on disease. News releases, prompted by the funds' recipients, assure the nation that cures are just around the corner. Most of us are no longer holding our breath in anticipation of the big events.

Looking beyond the pathological tissues to examine the many facets of psychology and physiology and determine cause and cure of disease has not been a popular thrust in medicine. We have been seduced by promises, too tempting, too easy, that germs and viruses were at fault for most of the ills of earth's creatures, and therefore they and their target organs should be the objects of interest. Furthermore, the behavior of human beings makes for complex, messy research, far more difficult to interpret than the behavior of single cells. To use Einstein's analogy, not many holes have been drilled through that thick end of the board.

Claude Bernard, the great French physician who is considered the founder of experimental medicine, expressed a similar concern as he observed the single-minded fervor of the microbe hunters during the mid-1800's. He and Pasteur carried on a controversy that spanned decades, with Bernard maintaining that illness hovered about continuously, but could not take root unless the terrain, i.e., the body, was receptive. He claimed the appropriate focus of study must therefore be the terrain itself. Pasteur, of course, along with Koch and others of his generation, was involved in the valiant attempt to identify and conquer the germ, and thereby rid humankind of disease. The story goes that on his death bed, having succumbed to one of the germs he'd tried in vain to irradicate, Pasteur conceded that Bernard, alas, was right. The microbe is nothing, the terrain everything.

Bernard taught that the study of physiology, and consequently pathophysiology, should in fact be quite reductionistic, at least at the onset. "When we come to analyze the complex manifestations of any organism, we should therefore separate the complex phenomena and reduce them to a certain number of simple properties belonging to elementary organisms; then synthetically reconstruct the total organism in thought, by reuniting and ordering the elementary organisms, considered at first separately, then in their reciprocal relations."[1] Always, Bernard's emphasis was on the *milieu interieur*, the amazing constancy of the internal environment, and the ability of that environment to protect and defend itself from the *milieu exterieur* in which the organism was situated.

Vaccination: Training the Immune System

All living things (including plants) have the potential for defending against disease. Most of the time, that defense network functions remarkably well to protect the organism from any invasion that disturbs the system. When it doesn't work—when it is for reasons of genetics, or too little or too much exposure to the offensive substances, or a lack of vitality caused by any number of reasons, including lifestyle—it can still be trained to attack with vigor and a highly selective aim. Immunization through vaccination is based upon this natural ability of the body to learn to defend itself. Vaccinations have provided medicines' most effective defense against disease. Early humans learned that a touch of a deadly infection left them with a strange power that protected them from subsequent encounters. The shamans, many of them, had come face to face with death before their vocation became apparent. No doubt their credibility was in part a function of some immunity gained through their illness.

Centuries ago, Chinese, Greeks, Turks, and Eastern Indians knew that smallpox, the dreaded scourge, the greatest killer of all, could be prevented by injecting bits of tissue or pus from a victim into a healthy person. In India, this grisly technique was considerably refined. Tissue donors were selected from persons who had a mild case of smallpox or who had already been vaccinated, or pus and tissues were dried for a year before being used as innoculation material. All these methods significantly decreased the risk of innoculation with a particularly deadly strain of the disease. In the early 1700's, when Lady Mary Wortley Montagu brought the Eastern methods to England, fully one-third of the adults bore the pitted remembrances of the disease. It was said that a mother dared not count her children until a smallpox epidemic had come and gone, because one of every fourteen children could be expected to die during the seige. The innoculations saved 99% of those treated. However, because of the occasional death, usually from unsterilized needles, vaccination was soon forbidden in England and in the Colonies as well.[2]

Lady Montagu's efforts were remarkably successful, and she could well have gone down in history as an angel of mercy, the savior of the children, a heroine for all time. However, Europe and England were not ready to be cured of smallpox until about one hundred years later. Then, Dr. Edward Jenner came upon the scene. A farm boy himself, he knew that milkmaids and farmhands were notorious for their unblemished complexions. He was also aware of the custom whereby rural parents would insist their children touch the udders of cows infected with cowpox. Far from being mere superstitious behavior, they were gaining immunity from smallpox. Their immune systems were being taught to react and to kill any invader that resembled cowpox, and that included the smallpox virus.

In 1798, Jenner published his successes in innoculating humans with fluid from infected cows, and within our lifetime we have seen the disease almost disappear from the face of the earth.

The ancient technique of using harmless or weakened microorganisms to stir up and fine tune the immune system is the principle of modern vaccination, and one that can be given credit for the giant leap in health over the last century. By 1910, vaccines had been developed for diphtheria, typhoid fever, and tetanus. And to date, polio, measles, mumps, rubella, whooping cough, and many forms of influenza are no longer a threat, thanks to the incredible ability of the immune system to learn new tricks.

What Do the Immune System and Dogs Have in Common?

The immune system naturally knows a tremendous amount about defense. Some of its information is genetically coded, some is absorbed from the mother during prenatal life and later from her milk. The white blood cells, the chief representatives of the immune system, have an uncanny ability to sort out friend from foe. After the enemy is identified, the means of destruction available to the white blood cells may include poisons, explosive techniques, strangulation, and immobilization. When the skills of the white blood cells go awry, autoimmune diseases, such as rheumatoid arthritis and multiple sclerosis, as well as infectious disease and cancer are possible.

What the immune system doesn't already know, or hasn't learned from vaccination, it may be able to learn in yet another way. Ivan Pavlov, the great Russian physiologist, is credited with establishing the basis for understanding how learning occurs in living things: dogs, humans, monkeys, and even single cells and cell populations.

Pavlov found that if he rang a bell and then offered meat to a dog several times, the dog would soon respond to the bell as if it were meat—by salivating, licking, and the usual doggy-type anticipatory responses to food. The pairing of one stimulus that naturally produced an eating response (the food), with one that did not (the bell), soon caused an association to be made between the two stimuli. The dog had learned to respond to the bell as if it were food.

This type of learning has dramatic consequences for human beings. Our bodies learn to respond to sounds of footsteps in the dark; they even learn to respond to thoughts of footsteps in the dark, as if they were really there. All the biochemical changes that happen during the real-life exposure can happen just as well during the fantasy. Thoughts of a passionate encounter can cause the same juices to flow as the encounter itself. A whiff of fresh lavender can bring forth a flood of memories of a loving grandmother's cozy room, along with feelings of relaxation and security.

It's been known for decades that heart rate and other so-called autonomic or involuntary functions could be trained to respond in various ways by setting up a situation such as that I've just described—by the paired association of a stimulus that normally produces such a change, and one that is neutral or does not. Robert Ader and his colleagues at Rochester Medical Center have conclusively demonstrated, study after study, that white blood cells, the body's army of defenders, can be trained in the same fashion as Pavlov's dog.[3] The gist of Ader's work, which was done with rats, is that when an immunosuppressive agent (some poisonous chemical that kills off white blood cells or otherwise inhibits their function) is paired with a harmless stimulus, such as a saccharin solution, the white blood cells learn to respond to the saccharin as if it were the poison itself. In fact, mortality rate is related to the amount of the harmless solution consumed—except that it is obviously no longer harmless as far as the conditioned white blood cells are concerned.

Work is currently underway to answer the more pressing question: Is the immune system capable of being activated or enhanced through the same procedure? The medical ramifications of the work have been demonstrated in a recent study using New Zealand mice.[4] These mice are typically used to study systemic lupus erythematosus (SLE), a serious autoimmune disorder that affects humans and is considered incurable. With most autoimmune disorders, as well as with cancer, cytotoxins (cell poisons) are occasionally a successful treatment. It is believed they halt the progressive multiplication of the offensive cells, which are more susceptible to the poison than the good, healthy cells. Ader and Cohen paired the cytotoxin cyclophosphamide with saccharin. The results indicated that the development of complications and mortality was retarded in the mice who had been conditioned to respond to the saccharin as if it were cyclophosphamide. It is conceivable that similar pairings might work with humans—pairing chemotherapy with a neutral substance, thereby training the body to respond to the neutral substance, and then using it intermittently instead of the toxic chemical. The therapeutic benefit would be served if some such scheduling could be devised so the toxic side effects of the drug could be reduced.

The Mind and Immunity

Stephen Locke and Mady Horning-Rohan published an annotated bibliography of over 1300 scientific articles, all written since 1976, relating to the mind's influence on immunity, and the associated neuroendocrine pathways.[5] Like all great discoveries, this work is coming simultaneously from hundreds of investigators, who, working independently, are arriving at a single-minded conclusion. The conclusion is that we can no longer think of immunity from disease as something that can be studied exclusively *in vitro,* in a test tube or under a microscope, or otherwise only outside the living organism. The immune system is smarter than that. It reacts to messages from the brain; it is, in fact, controlled by the brain.

Since 1950, work has been reported showing that the brain, particularly the structures involved in emotion (the hypothalamus and the pituitary gland), could be artifically stimulated to increase or decrease the activity of the immune system.[6] We conducted some of this work in our own lab, and found that when we mildly stimulated an area of the rat brain called the medial hypothalamus, the ability of the macrophages (literally the "giant eater" white blood cells) to consume "trash" in the blood was invariably diminished.[7] Other investigators report being able to increase the activity of the immune system with stimulation to other parts of the hypothalamus. Naturally this work is always conducted in the animal laboratory, and care must be taken when generalizations are made across species. However, for many areas of the brain, there is a remarkable correspondence of structure and function that is demonstrated by all mammals. The hypothalamus in the rat, for instance, looks and acts like the hypothalamus in a human. It is involved in temperature, eating, and drinking regulation; sexual behaviors and emotional responses; and in sending signals to the pituitary, the complex stalk-like gland that sits as kingpin over hormonal secretions. We can safely presume that in humans, as in rats, the hypothalamus is involved in immunity.

The mediation between the brain structures and the immune system was believed to happen through the endocrine system exclusively, until Dr. Karen Bulloch published her research in 1981. She surmised that since the thymus gland (which stimulates the production of T-cells) is crucial to the development of the hypothalamic-pituitary axis during the perinatal period, as well as to immune competence postnatally, there should be evidence of neural pathways connecting these structures. Consequently, she was able to identify neural projections from the spinal cord and the medulla to the thymus gland in both rats and mice, suggesting a role for these central nervous system structures in the regulation of thymic function.[8]

But so far, we have addressed only the so-called *lower* brain areas with regard to their role in immunity. The *mind*, on the other hand, is usually synonymous with the cortex itself. How can immunity be influenced by the many facets of the evolved mind: its language structure, its massive storage, its ability to reflect on and think about itself? Let us briefly examine both structure and function of the brain as it relates to this issue. (See Chapter 4 for more information on brain structures and imagery.) To begin, the hypothalamus (which, as we have mentioned, serves an important regulatory role in immune function) is intimately connected to the parts of the brain that are involved in emotion, i.e., the limbic system. The limbic system, in turn, forms a connecting network with the frontal lobes, which are the most evolved part of the cortex itself and believed to be critical for imagery and for planning for the future. The brain is really a mesh of interconnecting pathways, anyway, and activity in any one part affects the whole configuration in some way.

There is some evidence for cortical hemispheric specialization with regard to certain aspects of immunity. Bardos and his colleagues have shown that in mice, anyway, it is the left hemisphere of the cortex that controls the reactivity of the killer T-cells.[9] Some intriguing findings have been reported in humans by Geschwind and Behan, who have identified a relationship between left-handedness (i.e., right cerebral hemispheric dominance) and diseases of the immune system.[10] These studies, like most of the work in the field of psychoneuroimmunology, obviously need to be replicated to include broader samples and additional measures before any sound conclusions can be made. It is clear, though, that the cortex plays some role in the immune response.

The information presented above is integral to the thesis of this section, i.e., that the brain and the immune system are connected. It is of greater interest, however, whether actual behaviors or events that are known to be modulated by various brain areas can also be associated with changes in the immune system. For this information, we turn again to the literature on stress, recalling the pathways proposed in Chapter 4 involving the cortex, the limbic system, the hypothalamic-pituitary-adrenal axis, and subsequent inhibition of various healing mechanisms. During periods of high stress—such as space flight and recovery, school exams, and after long periods of sleeplessness—the immune system has been found to be significantly repressed. The year after a beloved husband or wife dies has always been recognized as a most vulnerable period when the bereaved may well follow along. Several studies have now demonstrated that the vulnerability has a very real basis. For a period of time after the death of a loved one, the immune system often loses its ability to react as well as it should—which creates an appropriate climate for heightened disease susceptibility. Furthermore, the identification of stressful antecedents prior to the onset of diseases involving the immune system has been a fertile area of research for two decades.

The critics of the psychoneuroimmunology research point out that, despite the above-mentioned findings, there have been no prospective studies where stressors are identified, the various components of the immune system are found to be suppressed, and immune-related disease is observed. In other words, we have evidence that stress precedes disease, and that stress inhibits the immune response, but no one has shown conclusively that the inhibited immune response associated with stress actually results in physical disease. The point is well taken, and certainly research in the future should take it into consideration. In any event, it is becoming more and more difficult to argue against the involvement of the brain in immunity, and consequently, in health.

Now the Good News

All this seems rather dismal so far: rats learning to get sick, and white blood cells forgetting their function in the face of stress. The information on how to use these same mental processes to get well has been much slower in coming. I dare say that most folks, and that includes scientists, believe that we make ourselves sick, but need to go to the doctor to get well. It is inconceivable that the human species could have come this far with the rather exclusive talent of making itself ill. That would scarcely be adaptive, or likely to encourage the survival of the fittest. Let's look at some of the evidence favoring the position that what we imagine and how we choose to live can have a positive effect on the immune system, as well.

Cancer as an Immune Disorder

We stand to learn much about the process of disease by studying the special cases: the anomolous individuals who manage to survive or return to health contrary to all of the soothsayers' grim predictions, and those who carry about with them a cushion of protection from the sea of microbes and the strains of living. The focus of this work is often on cancer. Cancer, in a sense, can be viewed as a disease of the immune system. Certain white blood cells, called T-cells, are targeted to identify and demolish any and all cancer cells they encounter in a most wonderful way. Picture a mighty midget, full of lethal toxins, stalking its prey. Finding the dreaded cancer cell, it thrusts itself inward like a missile, releasing its chemicals. Blisters form on the cancer cell, making it look as if it has been roasted on a hot grill. The blisters grow bigger and, within a millisecond, the cancer cell explodes into oblivion. The macrophages are called onto the scene as part of the clean-up team: they swell up, join forces, and head for the site of the destruction, programmed to digest any remaining pieces.

It is now believed that this process happens regularly in an otherwise healthy body. Any normal cell has the potential for losing its bearings and turning into an aberrant version of itself—one that knows only how to grow wildly, at the great expense of its host. Just as we often harbor the potential for strep and staph infections, we also have scattered malignant cells, which are being held in check by the T-cells and the macrophages. This is the surveillance theory of cancer, a theory that, while still controversial, has moved into some prominence. It is only when the prowling defenders fail to recognize or effectively kill the enemy that cancer cells are allowed to multiply into full-blown disease. Should cancer go into remission, it does so through this same process: the defending horde has successfully outflanked the tumor.

Spontaneous Remission

In the medical literature, there are numerous documented instances of so-called spontaneous remission from cancer. Eric Peper and Ken Pelletier conducted a computer search using medical library resources and obtained over 400 cases.[11] No doubt there are hundreds of thousands of such cases that remain the personal knowledge of health practitioners, but which go unpublished. "Spontaneous remission" is an odd term, meaning the disease went away without medical intervention, and for no known reason. It is one of those astonishing events in health, like the placebo effect, that attests to the ability of the body to heal itself. Since neither the placebo effect nor spontaneous remission involve "real" medicine, they have gone uncelebrated. The widespread instances of spontaneous remission pose questions, largely unanswered: Who are these people? What was going on in their lives? What happened to their immune system to cause such a dramatic change?

In looking at the wide variety of circumstances, several answers are plausible. Elmer and Alyce Green concluded that the only common factor among the 400 cases cited in the above-mentioned bibliography was a change of attitude prior to the remission, one which involved hope and positive feelings.[12] Some of the patients found a cure they believed in, whether it was the religious shrine at Lourdes or a fad diet. It has been my observation that the people who enter remission do so after latching onto a "cure" as true believers, ignoring dissuasion, defying the odds as well as medical opinion. I have no doubt that the numbers of cures reported by fringe practitioners are often inflated, but some do occur nevertheless. Apparently, anything can work if you believe in it enough, including wheat grass, Navaho sand paintings, healing waters, and chemotherapy. (There is no logical reason to believe the people who recover after having major poisons assault their system, such as in chemotherapy, are not also instances of spontaneous remission; they too can be regarded as having gotten well because of their attitude and in spite of the treatment.)

I have been privileged to hear of many instances of remission from all types of serious disease, from both expatients and physicians, alike. After each presentation of the material on the imagination and health, a handful of people stop me afterwards, and with a glow on their faces, obviously still feeling the wonderment of it all, will tell me the circumstances of their return to health. I hear again and again of self-discovered imagery procedures that were adopted out of sheer desperation. Fearing the consequences of the disease, or even of proposed treatment, the patients turned inward and began to work intensively with their minds.

A physical therapist told me of a time in her life when she was about to finish her master's degree and was suffering from massive uterine hemorrhage. All the usual treatments had been tried: hormones, dilation and curretage, bed rest. The only treatment left was hysterectomy—an unpleasant option since in the first place, it would probably keep her from graduating at her scheduled time; but more important, she was unwilling to face a life of childlessness at her age. She knew that she couldn't continue bleeding so profusely without serious consequences. She begged off her surgery for a week and went into seclusion. During this time she visualized a white light shining its healing rays into her uterus. At the end of the week, the bleeding had stopped completely. That was five years ago, and no similar problems had occurred since. She hadn't told her story to many people and, being in a medical profession, she was just a little embarrassed about the circumstances of her recovery. She was also unaware, even when I talked to her, that the white light had been used for centuries in all parts of the world in precisely the same capacity as she chose to use it.

About ten years ago, I participated in a health program at one of the metaphysical churches in a suburb of Los Angeles. The church was in a lovely garden setting, and had about it the special quality I've learned to associate with churches whose congregations are not afraid to think new thoughts. After the main presentations, the minister told a story only a few of his congregation had been privileged to hear. Several years before, he'd been plagued with a sore in his mouth. He went to his dentist, and then to a surgeon who biopsied the tissue and diagnosed it as a malignancy. The lesion was growing rapidly, and the recommended surgery would require removing a rather large portion of his jaw. He knew he must first seek out a healing place, and, searching his mind, he found it quickly in his memories of a visit to the sea wall on the coast of Oregon. Traveling there, he spent several days in deep meditation, concentrating exclusively, intensely, on the tissues in his mouth returning to normal. As a minister, his beloved career depended upon his ability to speak publicly. He'd developed a loyal congregation, and even a growing reputation for his television and radio work. The extensive surgical procedures would end all that. When he returned home, a second biopsy indicated no evidence of disease.

Dr. Stanley Krippner, a well-known scientist who has studied unusual healers, gave a seminar recently in Dallas. He was asked at the close of his presentation what single event most convinced him of the existence of special healing abilities. Instead of relating the names of any of the gifted healers he'd studied, he gave a personal example. Fifteen years previously, he'd had surgery for an abdominal problem. The incision failed to heal, and copious drainage from the wound indicated some internal problem was present. His physician was concerned and insisted he stay bedridden until the condition had cleared. Dr. Krippner called in one of his friends who had a talent for diagnosing illness. She said she believed the problem was with four of the stitches, which were either misplaced or had worked their way into an irritating position. He began to image the stitches coming out through the drainage tube. After two days, two double-knotted stitches popped out through the tube, and the incision healed promptly thereafter.

I am always touched by such stories. More than any research, they support the very special abilities of human beings to heal themselves when nothing else can. All of these cases could be regarded as spontaneous remission, some from more serious conditions than others. They were all conscious efforts to use the imagination, and the people involved all said it was some of the most difficult mental work they'd ever done in their lives.

Chemicals of Trust?

Spontaneous remission need not always follow a conscious attempt to use the imagination in a healing capacity. It may also follow events that lead not just to hope, but to the complete trust that good health is imminently to follow.

Bruno Klopfer told the poignant story of a man who heard that Krebiozen, a new wonder cure, was being tested at the hospital where he had been sent to die. He was initially turned down by the study committee as being too close to death to meet their criteria. Believing that Krebiozen was his last, his only hope, he convinced them to give him the experimental drug. Klopfer reported: "What a surprise was in store for me! I had left him febrile, gasping for air, completely bedridden. Now, here he was, walking around the ward, chatting happily with the nurses, and spreading his message of good cheer to any who would listen. Immediately I hastened to see the others who had received their first injection at the same time. No change, or change for the worse, was noted. Only in Mr. Wright was there brilliant improvement. The tumor masses had melted like snowballs on a hot stove, and in only these few days, they were half their original size! This is, of course, far more rapid regression than most radiosensitive tumors could display under heavy X-ray given every day. And we already knew his tumor was no longer sensitive to irradiation. Also, he had had no other treatment outside of the single useless 'shot.' Mr. Wright left the hospital practically symptom free, and even flew his own plane at 12,000 feet with no discomfort."[13]

Then, conflicting reports on Krebiozen's effectiveness were on the news. Mr. Wright's faith waned, and after two months of health, he returned to his original state. Figuring they had nothing to lose, his physicians administered a special "double strength" dose—or so they told him. Actually, it was pure water. Again, he returned to health. "Recovery from his second near-terminal state was even more dramatic than the first. Tumor masses melted, chest fluid vanished, he became ambulatory, and even went back to flying again. At this time he was certainly a picture of health."[14] It was another two months before the American Medical Association announced their findings: "Nationwide tests shows Krebiozen to be a worthless drug in treatment of cancer." Mr. Wright succumbed within days of the announcement.

Still other instances of spontaneous remission are found when lives are turned dramatically around, and the process of living is greeted with enthusiasm. The disease, itself, may have followed after a significant life change, one that caused life to lose meaning. The times in our lives when the chances of cancer, or even heart disease, enter into higher levels of probability are those years when major creative effort has ceased—the two years following retirement, or the period after the last child leaves the nest, regardless of one's age when that happens. When emotional and intellectual growth ceases, malignancy, a new and deadly growth process, takes over. For some, it is a reversible consequence if energy is poured into a renewed creative effort.

Larry LeShan, from his years of experience as a scientist/therapist, reports that there are basically three reasons a person gives for not wanting to die. Either (1) he or she fears the circumstances of death or dying—the pain, the unknown, the helplessness; or (2) he wants to live for others, to fulfill their demands and expectations; or (3) he wants to live his own life to "sing the unique song of his own personality."[15]

LeShan says, "For reasons I do not fully understand, the body will not mobilize its resources for either or both of the first two reasons. Only for the third will the self-healing and self-recuperative abilities of the individual come strongly into play. When individuals with cancer understand this and begin to search for and fight for their own special music in ways of being, relating, working, creating, they tend to begin to respond much more positively. . . ."[16]

Mobilizing the Defense

The body has specialized mechanisms for healing itself from most major disasters. Bones heal after being sparked with something known as bone morphogenetic protein (BMP), which induces fibro-blasts—bone cells that have healed as scar in the wake of a tumor or a bad fracture—to function as chondroblasts or normal cartilage-producing cells. The skin and other organs have evolved ways to constantly recondition themselves, or to continue to function in the face of damage. By the same token, the immune system is finely tuned to seek out and destroy all abnormal or foreign foes that invade the body, including cancer cells. Anything that doesn't look like "self" is relentlessly attacked.

In the instances of unusual recoveries, normal healing mechanisms such as these are responsible. No unique methods of healing beyond those normally prodded into action by the body in its own defense have ever been identified, regardless of source of cure. Alexis Carrel, a very astute observer of the scientific scene, reported on the so-called miraculous cures at Lourdes. These cures are carefully recorded by the Medical Bureau of Lourdes, and are available for inspection. Physicians are also invited to examine the patients as they come in and leave the healing shrine, and Lourdes itself has been the center for the multi-membered International Medical Association. Carrel stated that actually very few miraculous cures took place there. Those that did, though, followed a similar pattern: First, there was an acute pain, then a sudden sensation of having been cured. The visible wounds tended to heal in a normal way, except at a very fast rate. The miracle appeared to be chiefly characterized by an extreme acceleration of the normal processes of organic repair.[17]

Carrel's experience convinced him that medicine could progress only by studying the "inner mechanisms of endurance," the soundness of organs, and the individuals who either healed remarkably or were immune to infections, degenerative diseases, and the decay of senescence. He lamented the masking of organic lesions, and the mere administration of chemicals to the sick. "We have so far followed the easiest road. We now have to switch to rough ground and enter uncharted countries. The hope of humanity lies in the prevention of degenerative and mental diseases, not in the mere care of their symptoms. The progress of medicine will not come from the construction of larger and better hospitals, of larger and better factories for pharmaceutical products. It depends entirely on imagination, on observation of the sick, on meditation and experimentation

in the silence of the laboratory. And, finally, on the unveiling, beyond the proscenium of chemical structures, of the organismal and
mental mysteries."[18] This he said in 1935.

Chemicals of Recovery

As usual, the immune pathways that could account for disease and
destruction were investigated before the mechanisms for health.
These were found to include the activities of the hypothalamus,
the pituitary, and their associated glandular network. The connection between psychological stress and the inhibition of the immune
system was believed to occur as a result of excessive secretions of
hormones, particularly cortisone and cortisol, which have an anti-
inflammatory (or immunosuppressive) effect. We are permanently
indebted to the late Dr. Hans Selye for pioneering this important
work.[19]

Quite recently, evidence has been published that provides a potential link between positive mental processes and the acceleration of
the immune system. Several investigators have now shown that the
opiatelike chemicals found naturally in the human body, the endorphins and enkephalins, may have still another function in addition to producing euphoria and reducing pain: the enhancement of
the immune system. In a series of studies, the beta-endorphins increased the T-cells' ability to proliferate,[20] and enkephalins were
shown to invigorate the attack of T-cells against cancer cells.[21] The
enkephalins also increased the percentage of active T-cells.[22]

These magnificent chemicals are released automatically during times of pain and stress. It is also suspected that they are responsible for the natural feelings of ecstasy associated with multiple
events, including long-distance running, giving birth, and peak experiences of a spiritual nature. Just as losing a beloved may inhibit
the immune system, the physical changes that occur when one falls
in love may trigger recalcitrant immunology into action. The endorphins and enkephalins may be part of the biochemistry of the
hope and relief that accompanies a cure, any cure, and subsequently
leads to an often mystifying remission of illness.

This exciting work leads to the following four hypotheses concerning its relativity to the human condition:

(1) If the activities of the brain and the immune system
are intimately connected, then people with extremely efficient immune systems would be expected to be also different psychologically

or mentally from others whose immune systems were less capable of defending against disease.

(2) If mental activity and immune activity are connected, then the nature of the relationship can be demonstrated through a statistical association of the two factors.

(3) If mental phenomena are found to be related to immune activity, and the immune system is related to defense against disease, then either the mental phenomena or the nature of the immune system will correlate with the state of health.

(4) If there is a reciprocal relationship between mental activity and the immune system, such that either can cause a change or react to a change in the other, then the cause and effect relationship can be known by manipulating one circumstance and observing subsequent change in the other.

The most elemental tests of these hypotheses are reported in the following pages. The results will change the way medicine is practiced—not today, or next year, but soon. The changes will be facilitated more rapidly if nonscientists are able to critically evaluate the meaning of the research for their own lives. Even we who are scientists are finding that we must learn to speak an interdisciplinary language that spans medicine, psychology, immunology, biochemistry, and physics.

The research methods of the scientist are not sacred, but there are special conventions scientists must follow, which are not well known even to the well-educated nonscientists. It will help you in making your own decisions about the following research issues if I mention some of them.

First of all, the game of science is to stack the deck against oneself—over and over again. The situation is kept as pure as possible so the results obtained can be trusted to happen again under similar circumstances. For example, it is a common tactic to allow only those results to be considered significant that could have occurred only five or fewer times by chance alone out of a hundred studies (as determined by statistical analysis), and to throw out those that could have occurred by chance alone six or more times out of a hundred. This is the meaning of "significant" in research. It doesn't always make sense to throw out years of research effort just because this arbitrary definition of truth hasn't quite been reached, and important pioneering findings are often dismissed because of this convention. Yet, there is some comfort in knowing that only those results that are significant beyond a shadow of a doubt are reported as having significance, and wild conclusions are restrained.

There is also an unspoken trust among researchers, who assume the data are collected with integrity and reported honestly. Safeguards and watchdogs are built into research to assure this happens *most of the time*. Recently, scandals involving falsified results have been reported in fine institutions; still, dishonesty is relatively rare and we can probably believe most of what we read. The scientific method remains one of the best ways to openly and critically examine the structure and function of the human body/mind without delusion. The study of the brain and immune function could be carried just so far with introspection and debate alone.

Super Competence

The obvious way to study people with a peculiarly well-functioning immune system would be to take blood samples from thousands, select out those few who had stellar-quality white blood cells, and proceed to investigate them thoroughly. That is an obvious study, but, it is currently impossible. The state of the art in immunology is such that beyond the normal limits established for certain of the immune functions and the ability to detect some abnormalities, not much else is known regarding what constitutes high efficiency. We must, for the present, look elsewhere for information.

Certain populations who are exceptionally healthy are assumed to have a special protection from disease. Seventh Day Adventists and Mormons, for instance, have notoriously low incidences of heart disease and cancer. Members of the Unity church are seldom ill, and when they are, they recover rapidly, missing few days of work.[23] Other populations, such as the mentally retarded and emotionally disturbed, have a selective protection from cancer, as well as from autoimmune disorders such as rheumatoid arthritis,[24] but not from infectious disease such as upper respiratory problems.[25] The percentage of deaths from cancer for the mentally handicapped population is only about 4%, while 15–18% is the usual rate. And, as the mentally handicapped approach normal intelligence, their cancer rate increases also. A straw poll we conducted with two institutions that house the criminally insane, many of whom have acted out with heinous, unthinkable crime, also reveals that they are unusually protected from cancer, despite poor health habits, such as heavy smoking.

Superimmunity from killer diseases is apparent in certain communities where there are large numbers of very old people, such as the village of Vilcabamba in the Andean mountains of southern Ecuador, the land of Hunze in the Karakoram Range in Pakistani-controlled Kashmir, and Abkhazia in the Georgian Soviet Socialist Republic in the southern Soviet Union. These populations have been researched by Alexander Leaf, Sula Benet, Grace Halsel, and others.[26] Most agree that, while their ages may be somewhat exaggerated, the health, vigor and vitality of the elders remains highly significant and thoroughly documented, and that there are indeed exceptionally large numbers living past the age of 100, if not to 140, as claimed.

It is difficult to concoct any biological or psychological similarities among such diverse groups of individuals—the mentally handicapped, the natives of remote mountain regions, and devout and well-heeled church members. Probably there is none. Nutrition, genetics, geography, the avoidance of toxic substances, and the availability of modern medical care—the usual excuses for supreme health—are not common to all of the groups either. The criminally insane and the emotionally disturbed are often heavy smokers. Cigarettes are such prized items that they are used as reinforcement for good behavior. Reports on the aged folks describe them as daily imbibers of powerful native brew, and they usually smoke hand-rolled, locally-grown tobacco. The availability of modern medical facilities in the remote villages is nil. The Mormon emphasis on a pure diet, and the relatively simple but nutritious high-fiber, low red-meat diet of the aged groups may play some role. On the other hand, there is scarcely any nutritional benefit to being mentally handicapped. Institutional food has its shortcomings: little recognition is given for unusual nutritional needs of inhabitants, and the mentally retarded may require tube feeding for long periods.

The answers won't be simple. But consider, for a moment, the special, yet different, psychological issues among these people. The health of the Mormons and the Seventh Day Adventists may well come from the value that they place on good health habits. What of the value they likewise place on family life, on community? Might it not be conducive to health to feel a part of a network that would offer support—emotional, financial, spiritual, or whatever else you needed—for the rest of your life?

The situation is not so different for Unity and other New Thought church members, who place emphasis on good health within their religious teaching, and share the notion that each person is a part of

God and capable of attaining perfect health by living harmoniously with all of creation. These churches were founded with an emphasis on healing with the imagination, and believe perfect health is available through the power of conscious thought, and by imaging oneself as part of the perfect creation. They believe the mind and body and spirit are one entity, with the soul having dominion, and the body following the dictates of the mind. This metaphysical bent of the congregation, as well as the healing ministry of the pastor and trained teachers, surely also contributes to health. Unity and the other New Thought churches, unlike the more evangelical healing movements, do not particularly specialize in "cliffhanger" cures, but rather emphasize healthy living and disease prevention.

As far as the aged populations are concerned, immunity from disease is no doubt a combination of factors, including the gene pool in these isolated areas. All three groups are in rural mountain settings with an exceptionally high altitude, have low incomes, diets low in calories and animal fats, and lifestyles that demand a high level of physical activity. They appear to have unusual compensatory abilities that protect their health. Leaf reports that Dr. David Kakiashvili, a Georgian cardiologist, believes that the Abkhazians have all kinds of cardiovascular disease; but, he feels, the oxygen supply to the heart muscles is so well developed (presumably from the vigorous exercise), that if one artery gets pinched off from localized arteriosclerosis, there is still sufficient collateral circulation to enable the heart to function well. Therefore these folk may have few, if any, symptoms associated with the blockage.[27]

One of the most important facts, though, is that no one in any of these three populations ever retires or outlives their usefulness to society. Their self-image as living, viable, necessary human beings continues intact until death. The aged occupy a privileged position in these communities, and they continue to work at useful tasks within a close-knit family context as long as they live. They also believe in maintaining a happy marriage, often marrying soon after the death of a spouse, and continuing to be sexually active regardless of age. Their lifestyles ameliorate the two most vulnerable periods in the life of modern, Western society members: bereavement and retirement, the life passages associated with increased risk for disease and death.

And what about the mentally handicapped? How do they fit in? They have a selective immunity to cancer and perhaps the autoimmune disorders, such as rheumatoid arthritis, but not a generalized immunity. We can only speculate that there is a relationship between the diverse mental conditions of being retarded and emotionally disturbed, both of which indicate a lack of awareness of information from the environment, and immune disorders. Is it fear that's missing? Fear of disease itself? Is stress managed in some way that does not involve chemicals that inhibit the immune system? The criminally insane also have unusual methods for dealing with stress: They tend to attack the object of their discomfort, however illogically conceived, and immediately dissipate the flight or fight reaction. Anger is acted out, not harbored quietly until the chemicals eat their way into tissue.

All this raises more questions than answers. There is clearly more than one route for the mind to influence the immune system, and not all pathways are pretty. The most useful investigation might well be to determine whether the immune system could be consciously willed into action, since its activities are so entangled with the psyche anyway. What follows is an odyssey, undertaken to seek out evidence of that possibility.

The Exceptional Cancer Patients

The first step in the journey was taken with a small group of cancer patients, already diagnosed with "terminal" or Stage IV, widely metastatic, disease. This group included diagnoses of colon cancer with liver metastases, lung cancer with brain metastases, and breast cancer with lung and bone metastasis.[28] The life expectancy for these conditions, based on national tables, is one year or less. From twelve of those who had already outlived their predicted time by at least a year, a profile of the exceptional patient was generated. (This was based upon a series of psychological tests that included the Minnesota Multiphasic Personality Inventory, the FIRO-B, Locus of Control Scales, a sex role inventory, and an extensive medical and social structured interview.) The profile from the exceptional patients was then compared with profiles obtained from ten others with matched diagnoses who had succumbed at the time the tables predicted. The contrast in their psychological functioning was obvious. The patients who significantly outlived their expectancy were more creative, more receptive to new ideas, flexible, and argumentative. Often they were downright ornery. They had strong egos and expressed feelings of personal adequacy and vitality. Rather than seeking some outside source of emotional strength, they turned to their own inner resources. They sought out innovative medical treatment, refusing to accept the death sentence handed out with their diagnosis. In this sense, they were seen as using a form of denial—not denying the seriousness of their disease by any means, but denying that they would be victims.

These exceptional patients were unusual in many other ways. They were well-to-do, college educated, white, had more resources to turn to than the average patient, and they were all participating in the Simontons' cancer therapy groups, which at the time demanded high levels of psychological awareness. The group they were compared with were also part of this milieu, so the results cannot be attributed to those aspects of lifestyle just mentioned. But within that context, there was a profile associated with longevity, and hence, one can presume, a relatively stronger immune system.

A second type of exceptional cancer patient was identified from the research base established through the Cancer Rehabilitation Project, funded by the National Cancer Institute. The work was conducted at Parkland Memorial Hospital, the teaching facility for Southwestern Medical School in Dallas. There, the patients were racially mixed, poor and dependent upon the welfare system, and had few, if any, psychological resources to use to cope with serious disease. Some, through a far different set of adaptive mechanisms than those used by the Simonton patients, managed to stabilize and function very well in their daily activities. The majority had been given a diagnosis of metastatic breast cancer, lung cancer, or gastrointestinal cancer. These patients were administered similar tests as those described above, but often the tests had to be modified or read to them, because most could not read beyond the third-grade level.

Here, the profile of the exceptional patients was one of turning outward, looking for an external resource to give them renewed strength. Sometimes this was a person, often church or a job. The existence of a good relationship with their husbands was extremely important to the women's progress. The women in the study were from matriarchal subcultures where intact marital relationships were rare, and any long-term marriage would be regarded as an unusually stable situation. Sociability was also important to their well-being—a factor in opposition to the results of the tests of the first group of patients, whose survival was related to turning inward to self.

In both studies, the long-term survivors and short-term survivors were not substantially different on any physical or demographic characteristics. The breast cancer patients at Parkland had all received basically the same treatment: surgery followed by a mild form of chemotherapy. The Simonton patients had received the appropriate treatment for their particular disease—whatever that might have been at the time. There are no miracles in cancer treatment; there is nothing known that would consistently trigger exceptional recovery or the lengthy survival that some of these patients experienced.

After this work was published, other investigators reported similar findings. Leonard Derogatis and his colleagues, for instance, found that long-term survivors within a sample of metastatic breast cancer patients evidenced more emotion such as anxiety, depression, and guilt than did the short-term survivors. Also related to survival was a poorer adjustment to the illness, as perceived by the treating oncologists, and a significantly poorer attitude toward their physicians. The short-term survivors, on the other hand, were characterized by lower levels of hostility and higher levels of positive mood.[29]

The long-term survivors, the exceptional patients who shook their fists in the face of death, were fighters. Should we be surprised that their immune systems fight? Or that passive persons, the real sweethearts who die before their time, have immune systems that are also passive?

A San Francisco psychiatrist who has worked with cancer patients for a long time believes that the patients who do well already knew how to fight before they were diagnosed. I think he is absolutely correct, although no one has ever studied the issue systematically. People who have been in difficult straits and escaped from them have learned to rally their defenses and test their resources. They have already identified a support system. If you don't already know how to fight, learning how when you're scared, sick, and in pain may be next to impossible. Those who have been defined as passive patients seem bewildered that the same virtues that succeeded for them in the past—kindness, graciousness, a giving constitution, a cheerful outlook—don't work in the struggle against disease.

An adult's immune system typically doesn't have an automatic defense targeted specifically toward any newly encountered disease. The defense is only learned by a brush with the disease itself, or from a vaccination that teaches the immune system to respond appropriately. The fighters, too, have been inoculated in a special way.

Mind and Chemistry

The next level of investigation involves the identification of what, if any, biochemical differences might be associated with the psychological phenomena of exceptional recovery.

In 1975, when we proposed researching the relationship between blood chemistry and mental events, the only interested funding source was the Institute for Noetic Science, an organization that had been primarily concerned with parapsychology. They awarded $50,000 for the study to the Simontons' Cancer Counseling and Research Center in Ft. Worth, with half of the sum designated to a well-known cellular biologist who was to conduct electron microscope studies of the white blood cells. Within five years, the *Zeitgeist* had changed sufficiently to allow for replication of the work in major university settings with more conventional financial backing, demonstrating an unusually rapid shift in consciousness. All the work is still viewed suspiciously by the conservative scientific establishment, but at least it's now on the fringe, which I consider a distinct movement toward the inner sanctum of acceptance.

The research we conducted with the Noetics grant teetered constantly on the brink of disaster, with loss of important data, funding uncertainties, and interpersonal strife—features I've come to associate with the more worthwhile projects. Seven tubes of blood were drawn from each of 126 patients, and at the same time, they were asked to complete a full battery of psychological tests requiring about three hours of their time. This was an unusually generous offering from these people, 90% of whom had been diagnosed as having Stage IV, or widely metastatic, "terminal" cancer. The tests could not easily be repeated or recovered if lost. Most of the blood was designated to be sent several hundred miles away to the cellular biologist, and for an endless number of reasons, the early shipments were delayed until the blood was no longer usable.

It was then decided to conduct whatever analyses were possible with local laboratory facilities to salvage the study. The blood chemistry and hematological measures we included at that point were a complete blood count, cholesterol, cortisol, free fatty acids, acid and alkaline phosphatase, lactic dehydrogenase, and several others. It was a fortunate decision. The state of the science of cellular biology, using the electron microscope as an assay tool, was such that no possible statistical association could ever have been made between the pictures of the immune system and the psychological scales. At best, certain immune components could be identified as "unusual," but the question, "How do the immune system and psychological factors interrelate?" could not be answered. In most ways, the precision of measurement of psychological factors far surpassed the biological phenomena.

The first step, though, was taken by using those blood chemistry values that could be given a numerical value and for which some "normal limits" were known. Those were compared with psychological scales that had also been studied long enough to prove with some certainty that they were reliable and actually measured what they were supposed to measure. Some of these tests were mentioned previously in connection with the exceptional patients' profile. Added to the battery was what turned out to be impetus for future research, and the most important of all the research findings: an analysis of the patients' images of cancer, of treatment, and of the immune system itself. Again and again, the significant findings spiraled around the images as the most important predictors of health. The results held true even in the medical school/teaching hospital, where patients could scarcely have had the intellectual awareness that images had provided most of the medical knowledge through recorded history, or that they formed the basis for a controversial kind of cancer therapy.

The statistical treatment that was required for the large amount of data collected was extremely sophisticated. Furthermore, the complexity of the results has kept the impact of the findings obscure. Dr. G. Frank Lawlis, one of a handful of psychologists who understood how to analyze such data (in fact he had written a textbook on the subject), was introduced to me when the data were collected, but the funds for the requisite elegant treatment and computer time were not available. As a new faculty member at North Texas State University, he obtained a grant, computer time, and the assistance of a computer programmer. The results of the analysis have been reported in a statistical journal—the only one that would, at the time, consider the soundness of the design and analysis, and overlook the fact that rather astounding and controversial conclusions would inevitably be drawn from the findings, conclusions that would call into question the whole approach to the treatment of cancer.

The gist of the analyses was as follows: Three personality profiles emerged that associated both the blood chemistry and the psychological factors. The components of those profiles appear in Appendix F. The first profile was called *resignation*, based on both the negative, depressed aspects of the bloodwork and the psychological variables of these particular patients. The second combination of blood chemistry and psychological variables was called *nondirected struggle*. These patients appeared dissatisfied and worried, struggling and anxious; but their conflict was without direction. The blood profiles for both of these groups were consistent with a diagnosis of macrocytic hypochromic anemia. The third profile, the most positive, we called *purposeful action*. Both blood and psychological factors were consistent with a directed attempt to fight off disease. The blood indicated a compensatory anemic reaction to hemoglobin deficiency, with a relatively higher white blood cell count that could be interpreted as more antibody availability. Psychologically, these patients were unlikely to decompensate in the face of stress, were self-sufficient, and exhibited a belief in their own ability to control their situation.

The overriding conclusion was that, within the sample studied, there were three differing psychological profiles that appeared to represent a sort of continuum, starting from an attitude of giving up, extending to an attitude of ambivalent struggle, and finally reaching to include a purposeful and positive striving to overcome the disease. These were related to distinctive hematological profiles. Only in the most positive profile was the immune system seen to be enhanced.[30]

Prediction of Status of Disease

There was no question that a relationship existed between the blood components and the psychological scales, but exactly what that might mean in terms of the outcome of the disease had to be investigated in yet another way. The data had to be condensed into workable, understandable chunks, using what is called a "factor analysis." Then, those chunks that fell naturally together were used to determine two things: the relationship between blood, psychology factors and state of disease at (1) the time of testing; and (2) at a two-month follow-up. Present disease status was determined by scaling the most recent treating physician's report, with a "4" indicating significant new tumor growth; "3" no new tumor growth; "2" tumor(s) regression; and "1" no evidence of disease. For follow-up, a "5" was added to indicate the patient had died.

These categories were then correlated with the factors that had been identified. Briefly, the present disease was correlated with five factors, three of them blood variables, and two psychological (Figure 6-1). One blood factor was composed exclusively of white blood cells, and the second, primarily of cortisol and cholesterol, hormones associated with the stress response. Also associated with this second blood factor was the third, an enzyme called acid phosphatase, believed to be one of the poisons used by the immune system. Psycho-

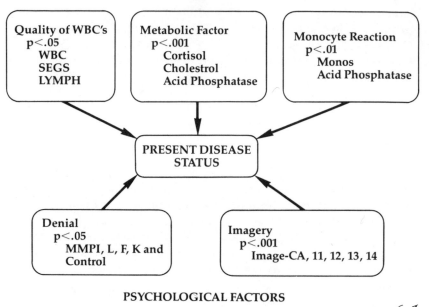

BLOOD FACTORS

Quality of WBC's
p<.05
WBC
SEGS
LYMPH

Metabolic Factor
p<.001
Cortisol
Cholestrol
Acid Phosphatase

Monocyte Reaction
p<.01
Monos
Acid Phosphatase

PRESENT DISEASE
STATUS

Denial
p<.05
MMPI, L, F, K and
Control

Imagery
p<.001
Image-CA, 11, 12, 13, 14

PSYCHOLOGICAL FACTORS

6-1

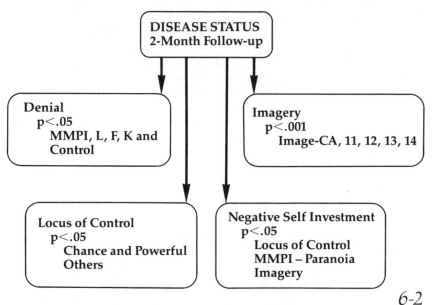

PREDICTABILITY OF PSYCHOLOGICAL FACTORS

DISEASE STATUS
2-Month Follow-up

Denial
p<.05
MMPI, L, F, K and
Control

Imagery
p<.001
Image-CA, 11, 12, 13, 14

Locus of Control
p<.05
Chance and Powerful
Others

Negative Self Investment
p<.05
Locus of Control
MMPI – Paranoia
Imagery

6-2

logically, a factor of denial (which came from the MMPI scales) was related, but by far the most significant correlate was the imagery—the patient's images of cancer, treatment and the immune system, as measured in a highly specific fashion. Again, these five factors were associated with state of disease, and served well in a diagnostic framework.

The ticklish issue was whether or not any of the factors actually preceded the change in disease, in which case they become prognostic of future outcome, if not causative. Those factors predicting disease status at two-month follow-up appear in Figure 6-2. None of the blood work was predictive. Apparently, the blood only reflects a current state of physiological functioning. The blood factors, particularly those associated with the immune system, are in a constant state of reaction to previous events, so interpreting the analysis is like looking through a rear-view mirror: You can see where you've been, but not where you're going.

The psychological factors that were predictive of future events were those related to denial, a sense of control, negative self-investment—and once again, the most predictive was the imagery. So it seems that while the blood factors were merely reacting to history, the psychological factors were predictive of the future outcome.

This work has been beautifully and ambitiously extended by Robert Trestman who used additional blood and hematological tests, as well as an expanded psychological assessment, and medical history variables.[31] Trestman came to similar conclusions regarding the relationships among the many measures. He also found that the imagery was a singularly powerful and independent factor, and that it tapped something that was untouched by other psychological tests. The relationships among blood work, psychological factors, and immunity are multiple and complex. It's possible that Trestman and we both exhibited a streak of genius in choosing the measures that we did, since we were able to identify so many relationships. (I'll admit they weren't exactly pulled out of a hat.) It's more probable, though, that all aspects of the body/mind are so entangled that eventually, as our measuring devices become sensitive enough, we'll find everything is connected to everything. Each aspect of human functioning affects every other aspect, but in greater or lesser measure. As for the immune system, the imagination has consistently proved to have the most directive influence. It has, as is said in the words of researchers, "contributed the most to the variance."

The Imagination, Quantified

The imagination, like love, has been regarded as sacred ground, too intimate, too holy, to be dissected by the impersonal knife of science. It was also regarded as too remote, since it couldn't be felt, smelled, or otherwise observed through the senses. This was before computers were built that allowed impossibly long computations to be carried out with ease. The following system for analyzing cancer imagery has become a prototype for subsequent studies dealing with arthritis, diabetes, pain, and discomfort/disease in a projective test called the "Image CA," after the studies discussed above suggested that the images were the most important factor in disease response.[32]

The patients' imagery reflected their attitudes about the disease and treatment, as well as any belief they might have in their innate ability to overcome the illness (via the immunological system or other properties of natural recovery.) For cancer, the latter typically was represented by the white blood cells. Often the attitudes assessed by virtue of the imagery were at odds with what the patients said they believed—indicating that the powerful concepts were not always to the conscious fore.

Imagery is assessed first by having a person get in a comfortable position, preferably lying down, and listen to tape-recorded relaxation instructions. There is good evidence that imagery flows best when the motor system is not actively competing for the brain's attention, and when the person is in a prone position.[33] Then, a very brief type of education is provided to inform the patient of the disease process, of how treatment might be working to the patient's advantage, and finally, the idea of host defense, or the immune system, is presented. The listener is then advised to imagine these three factors in action. The imagery is guided, but not programmed in the sense of suggesting to people that they imagine the cancer cells or the white blood cells as looking like anything in particular. This is their choice. Those ideas that spring from the depths of their psyche are drawn by the patient, and then described in an interview, structured with such questions as, "Describe how your cancer cells look in your mind's eye" and "How do you imagine your white blood cells fight disease?"

The interview protocol, plus the drawings, are then scored on the basis of fourteen dimensions that were determined by an earlier data analysis that quantified the components of the imagery. The dimensions include the vividness, activity, and strength of the cancer cell; vividness and activity of the white blood cells; relative comparison of size and number of cancer and white blood cells; strength of the white blood cells; vividness and effectiveness of medical treatment; choice of symbolism; the integration of the whole imagery process; the regularity with which they imaged a positive outcome; and a ventured clinical opinion on the prognosis, given the previously listed thirteen factors. All the dimensions are readily scorable on a "1" to "5" scale (from negative to positive), and those who rate the imagery tend to reach a high level of agreement about what score to give (i.e., the test is reliable). The scores, weighted by virtue of their total contribution to the total score (again, thanks to the miracles of computers and statistical analysis), are summed up and a total imagery score is obtained.

The format for the test was derived after listening to about 200 cancer patients talk about their imagery, and noting which issues seemed to foretell a change in prognosis. Normalization studies were conducted—one with 58 patients from the Cancer Counseling and Research Center and another with 28 patients who were attending the Cancer Rehabilitation Clinic at Parkland Memorial Hospital. A third study was conducted with men with cancer of the larynx who were participating in a National Cancer Institute project at the University of Texas Health Science Center, San Antonio.[34]

The total scores were found to predict with 100% certainty who would have either died or shown evidence of significant deterioration during the two-month period, and with 93% certainty who would be in remission. Remember, the scores are just a numerical shape put on the imagination—it was the images themselves that so accurately predicted the future. In other studies, the imagery was used to predict rehabilitation outcome, such as the ability to learn esophageal speech following laryngectomy, and the regaining of physical strength, range of motion in the arms, and return to daily activities following mastectomy.

What the patients' imaginations predicted were the dramatic changes that would occur within a short period of time. These results are often confusing to people who haven't witnessed the erratic course of cancer. Tumors can change as rapidly as nightblooming flowers, growing, shrinking, perhaps changing shape. People diagnosed with Stage IV cancer may be living active lives with few symptoms and no pain, or they may be bedridden; and they can move from one of these conditions to the other, and back, within days. Some of the changes are reactions to the treatment, but many are a function of the waxing and waning of the disease and the immune components. None of the patients in the studies mentioned so far were hospitalized when the original data were collected; in fact, most were on minimal pain medications, alert, active, and able to get to the clinics by themselves.

Trestman found twelve correlations between the images of cancer and of the white blood cells (as measured by the Image CA) and hematology and blood chemistry measures. When he added his own imagery dimensions, which involved the color of the cancer and the metaphorical qualities of the selected images themselves (instead of what the patients say *about* the images), such as dangerousness, overall strength and actual activity, another eleven correlations were noted. Only about one significant correlation would be anticipated solely by chance. (See Appendix G for list of correlations.) Trestman's analysis of color was interesting: Thirteen of the fourteen people with "good" status described their cancer as red or black, while eight out of the eleven with relatively poorer status described their cancers as lighter colors. (Trestman's subjects were neither extremely ill, nor were any in total remission, although all had been diagnosed as Stage IV.)

Symbols as Symptoms

In order to make sense of the imagination as a diagnostic specialist, some common factors must be identified. Otherwise, imagery remains such a highly individualized matter that there is no purpose in analysis. The Image CA did extract common factors in terms of the *features* of the symbols (i.e., size, activity, numbers, etc.), but the *kind* of symbol chosen was not invariably predictable of outcome. Trestman also analyzed the metaphorical quality of the symbols, as mentioned above, but his subjects were not so diverse culturally as ours. The symbols will remain characters in a rich and unique drama, depending upon the cultural context to gain meaning, and reflecting each person's developmental history. Their great value to the therapist lies precisely there. (I should state, though, that there are intriguing trends apparent throughout the symbols of all cultures that indicate a thread of collective ideation.)

Several years ago, in New York City, we presented a training workshop on the administration of the Image CA, designed as continuing education training for the American Psychological Association. A very disgruntled woman, who we found out later was a "workshop junkie" with a personal agenda, managed to enroll. To the great distraction of the other attendees, she demanded vociferously and repeatedly that we cease the teaching format and tell her quickly what to image to get rid of her cancer. "Quick, tell me," she said, "I don't have all day." I wish it could be that simple.

As researchers, we could evaluate extremely accurately the symbolic intent of the images of the white, college-educated patients. But beyond certain basic themes, we were abominable at understanding the symbology of the Mexican/American and Black charity patients at Parkland Hospital. Even the designation of "white" blood cell was commented upon as having some racial implication. One or two would laugh, and say, "I think I'll make mine black." One woman drew her cancer in the shape of a lemon, and colored it yellow, "because it reminds me of my husband," she said.

The images evoked are a broad collection of creative effort. The procedure opened up realms of communication, and allowed the patients to tell their stories in a new way, as never before. As they talked and drew the products of their imagination, I could travel the difficult road of life-threatening disease with them, glimpsing for an instant their metaphors, touched by the knowledge that all their life's energy was now beamed onto this moment, this disease. What power the archvillain cancer has, to be able to grab the human psyche and shake its foundations.

The symbols that so quickly emerged into consciousness when the questions were asked were as much a part of the patients' lives as the symptoms were part of the disease. The symptoms were symbols, the symbols symptoms. (The two words have essentially the same meaning—a concrete or tangible object that stands for an intangible idea.) And they both deserve equal respect for influencing the course of lives. The cancer was viewed as the enemy invader, occasionally the trickster, sometimes the battle scar from a wasted, broken life. The immune system was synonymous with the patients' own self-concept. When it was imaged as strong and pure, it overcame disease.

I will discuss the few patterns that did emerge, although reluctantly, because they mean less in terms of prognosis than the dimensions of the Image CA. Archetypal figures who fought for God and country and who were protectors of their people, such as Sir Richard, the knights of the Round Table, and the venturesome Vikings, were nearly always associated with a positive outcome. Animals with killer instincts such as sharks, bears, and mean dogs were sometimes, but not always, associated with good responses. Some people tried to force these images because they thought they were the most likely killers, but at the same time, they got disgusted with the gore.

Very poor responses were associated with vague, weak, amorphous symbols for the immune system such as snowflakes or clouds. More often than not, those with the worst prognosis just couldn't draw or describe anything at all related to the immune system, but had vivid images of their cancer. The cancer images tended to be more biologically correct, and hence, less symbolic than the white blood cells. A truly poor outcome was forecast when the cancer cells were seen as immutable, grasping, or ineradicable, when symbolized as lumps of coal, crabs, ants, or submarines; a better outcome was likely when they were described as weak animals or even as the actual cells as one might view them under a microscope. Interestingly enough, the insect images are a grim omen of disease in the shamanic system as well.[35]

The current thinking expressed among health professionals working with cancer is that much of the early work on imagery has placed too much emphasis on anger, and on killing and hating cancer; it is felt that a better prognosis might be obtained if one could learn to accept the cancer as part of oneself. That, too, might be an individual matter, although the evidence from Derogottis' and our work suggests that a better physical outcome can be expected when acceptance and adjustment to the cancer is the poorest. Only in the charity clinic patients could we find evidence that the existence of a symbiotic, positive relationship with the cancer was related to better physical health.

War on Warts

Images provide messages that are understood by the immune system. They link conscious thoughts with the white blood cells in such a way that the appropriate combinations and numbers come rushing forth to perform in ways that not even the most knowledgeable immunologist could command. Lewis Thomas makes this point in a charming essay on a most unlikely subject: the wart.[36]

The wart is a bunch of cells infected by a virus. Warts appear overnight, achieve the most permanent of appearances, and then disappear as quickly as they came. "And they can be made to go away by something called thinking, or something like thinking. This is a special property of warts which is absolutely astonishing, more of a surprise than cloning or recombinant DNA or endorphin or acupuncture or anything else currently attracting attention in the press."[37]

The power of the imagination makes warts go away, regardless of whether the trigger is called hypnosis, or suggestion, or the magic of an old woman who makes you turn around three times in the closet and then tells you they'll be gone in a week.

My own daughter once had warts, so many of them that the dermatologist said freezing them or surgery would leave too many scars on her little hands. He said, "Maybe they'll go away. Try some magic." We did, and they didn't. By then it was time to go visit her grandparents for the summer. What a treat was in store. They were keeping a big white horse for her to ride as long as she was there. A ten-year-old's veritable dream come true, and no one had ever seen her happier. After the first day, the wart infestation disappeared completely. She knew instantly that the horse was responsible. By some mechanism, her joy had interacted with her immune system in such a way that it recognized and attacked the viral invasion.

"But any mental apparatus that can reject a wart is something else again. This is not the sort of confused, disordered process you'd expect at the hands of the kind of Unconscious you read about in books, out at the edge of things making up dreams or getting mixed up on words or having hysterics." Among its accomplishments, Thomas says, this Person or Tenant in charge of healing must be a surgeon, a skilled engineer and manager, a chief executive office, and a cell biologist of world class. If we just knew exactly how a wart was thought away, he says, we would then know the identity of the biochemical participants in tissue rejection, and even the nature of certain diseases. "Best of all, we would be finding out about a kind of superintelligence that exists in each of us, infinitely smarter and possessed of technical know-how far beyond our present under-standing."[38]

It all seems so uncertain—having to go look up a hypnotist, or bury a rag at the crossroads by a full moon, or find a source of intense pleasure. What if you just directed the white blood cells to go kill the thing off? Well, as Thomas says, we just don't know which ones to call up. Who knows whether it's the T-cells or the B-cells; or if it is the T-cells, which ones? The killers? The suppressors? Maybe it's just the garden variety scavengers, the neutrophils and the macrophages. Suppose we did know? Could the superintelligence then sort among them and pick the recruits? Let's examine that possibility.

White Blood Cells

The neutrophils and the lymphocytes are the heroes of this story. First let's look at the neutrophils. These are white blood cells that are given life in the bone marrow, and constitute about 65% of the total white blood cell population. They are chiefly responsible for fighting infections, and are kept busy on a day-to-day basis, circulating about, looking for bacteria and other trash that doesn't belong in the body. They are executioners, par excellence. When chemicals are released at the site of an injury, the neutrophils prepare for attack by changing shape so they can better get through the vessel walls to do their deadly business. They then adhere to the walls of the capillaries, which have become sticky just for that purpose, and extend a small foot (called a *pseudopod*, which means, and looks just like a "false foot") through any convenient gap. Slithering their way out of the blood stream, they move toward the offender, and begin the process of destroying the intruders, which is called *phagocytosis*. The engulfment and digestion is accomplished when the neutrophil sends its cytoplasm flowing around the foreign particle, and then isolates it in a sac (a *phagosome*, it's called). Enzymes are then shot into the sac, and the intruder is destroyed. The enzymes eventually destroy the neutrophil, too, but since about 100 billion are produced a day, the loss is normally insignificant. This is only the beginning of the grand march; the neutrophils are followed by flank after flank of specialized attackers. Think of the neutrophils as the first line of defense, constantly active even in—or especially in—a healthy person.

B-cells and T-cells are both called lymphocytes, because they circulate through the lymph fluid. Both are targeted to respond only to certain microorganisms, and both are given their life in the embryonic bone marrow. The T-cells then migrate to the thymus, where they are energized for action. (Where the B-cells are thusly processed remains a mystery.) The T's usually wait in the lymphatic tissue, and are transported through the clear lymph fluid when it is time to deal with hostile organisms. There are actually at least three kinds of T-cells: the *killers*, whose speciality is killing viruses and foreign tissue with potent chemicals; the *helpers*, who assist the B-cells in going after their highly specific targets; and the *suppressors*, who serve a regulatory function, perhaps keeping the immune system from going wild and attacking self as well as nonself. The killer T's are known to be involved in the defense against cancer; the suppressor T's in the prevention of autoimmune breakdown. The B-cells, on the other hand, create proteins called antibodies that can identify a specific invader and start the complicated process of its destruction.

The next three studies, some of the most advanced research in science today, all involve the control of either the neutrophils or the lymphocytes with a mental process. The first study uses hypnosis; the second, biofeedback-assisted relaxation training; and the third, imagery specifically geared toward the control of a single function of the neutrophil. These are investigations that I have been privileged to follow for some time, and they have altered my own thinking about the power of the imagination. The methods of all the researchers are unimpeachable, and they have run the studies again and again. The work could only have come about with cooperation between basic and behavioral scientists.

Hypnosis and the Immune System

Dr. Howard Hall, a young psychologist working at Pennsylvania State University, together with his colleagues, Drs. Santo Longo and Richard Dixon, used hypnotic techniques with healthy subjects and then measured the effects on immune function.[39] Before we examine the study, first let me make a comment on hypnosis.

Most hypnotists will agree that hypnosis is contingent upon the imagerial system. Even the induction instructions given by therapists who use hypnosis are often identical to those given by therapists using guided imagery. In the past, though, hypnosis tended to allow less leeway for the subjects to create their own images, and more reliance was placed on the hypnotist's ability to program whatever mental images were apfrom for the desired outcome. While many hypnotists still maintain an authoritarian style, many others do not, particularly those who teach self-hypnosis or autohypnosis. Therapists may either show strong allegiance to notions of guided imagery or hypnosis, or they may not. Both groups have founded their own organizations and conduct training.

Even though the differences are erudite, I think they're important. The mystique of the traditional, authoritian hypnotist, the belief that he or she has special mental powers, and the programming of the mental images, may be much more effective for some patients. In many ways, the old-style authoritarian hypnosis is more like the techniques of the shamans than the more permissive educational format of guided imagery. The good shamans, like good hypnotists, would know what images to program, since they are quite specific to the culture and described in ancient songs and portrayed in art. On the other hand, a person may need the freedom to adopt his or her own symbol system in order to gain access to the hidden reaches of the immune system. That's only a supposition and a study for the future. For now, hypnosis fits well within the context of healing with the imagination, however practiced.

For the study, Hall and his coworkers recruited twenty healthy male and female volunteers, ranging in age from twenty-two to eighty-five. A prehypnosis baseline record of lymphocyte function was made. Then the subjects were hypnotized with a relaxation procedure, and asked to imagine a calm scene. The experimenter then counted to twenty to deepen the relaxation, and told the subjects to imagine themselves floating down on a cloud. Then they were asked to visualize and feel their white blood cells increasing in number and swimming like powerful sharks attacking weak and confused germs. This continued for five minutes. The subjects were told the sharks would continue defending them even when they weren't thinking about it. They were given written and verbal information on self-hypnosis, and advised to practice twice daily for a week. In addition to the prehypnosis baseline test, blood was again drawn after the first session, and once again after the second session, one week later. All subjects were tested for their ability to be hypnotized with the Stanford Hypnotic Susceptibility Scale.

Several analyses were performed on the blood, including total white cell count, total lymphocyte count, total T-cell and B-cell counts, and tests of the function or reactivity of the T-cells and B-cells. To assess the effect, the subjects were divided into an older group and a younger group (over and under the age of fifty). On three of the tests involving the stimulation of the T-cells with a mitogen, the younger group showed a statistically significant increase in immune functioning at one week after the procedure. The older group did not, a finding potentially attributed to the suppression of immune function that is normal with aging. (However, these conclusions are an artifact of statistics: for the younger group, the results could have happened only 5 times out of 100 by chance, and therefore were deemed significant. For the older group, they could have happened only 10 times out of 100 by chance; therefore, as a good researcher, by convention, Hall had to throw the results out, even though there was substantial evidence to suspect some influence occurred.)

The researchers felt their most important findings, however, concerned the relationship between immunity and hypnotizability. Based on the Stanford Scale, high and low hypnotizable groups were formed. A significant increase in lymphocyte count was noted one hour after the hypnosis procedure, but for the high hypnotizable subjects only. The elevation was not apparent after a week for either group.

Biofeedback-Assisted Relaxation and Immune Function

For her doctoral dissertation, Dr. Barbara Peavey studied the effect of a biofeedback-assisted relaxation program on immune function. (In 1984, the paper describing the study was presented to the Biofeedback Society of America's annual meeting by her and coauthors Drs. G. F. Lawlis and A. Goven, and was recognized as the most noteworthy scientific achievement of the year.)[40]

First, Dr. Peavey collected a group of sixteen people who were under high levels of stress and also had low levels of immunity, as measured by white blood cell counts and a test of the ability of the neutrophils to phagocytize or ingest debris. Half were assigned to a control group, half to the biofeedback program. These latter subjects were given instructions on biofeedback; baseline levels of relaxation were obtained using the biofeedback equipment; and following this, individual hour-long sessions were held twice a week. The training included home practice with cassette-recorded relaxation exercises, and specific information on stress. The subjects were trained with both EMG (a muscle monitor) and temperature biofeedback until they had reached a level that previous researchers had determined was related to a state of relaxation. These procedures are well recognized and widely employed among biofeedback therapists for training people to relax and learn to reduce the physical effects of stress. Blood samples were collected initially to identify the subjects, as mentioned above, again at the beginning of the biofeedback-assisted relaxation sessions, and after each subject had met the criteria for relaxation.

When the bloodwork on these subjects was compared to their own pretreatment tests and to the control group who had not received any treatment, their neutrophils were found to function significantly better following treatment. There were no differences in numbers of white blood cells, which indicates the effect was related to function only. Nothing was said to these subjects about the immune system, nor was the purpose of the study discussed. However, when these highly stressed individuals learned to relax under the careful conditions that Dr. Peavey employed, there was a direct but selective effect on immunity.

Other investigators have found that relaxation alone is not a sufficient condition to change the immune system, but that some imagery or visualization procedure is also required.[41] However, in these subsequent studies only one session of relaxation training was offered. This would not be likely to have any immediate consequences, since often many sessions are required before the relaxation response is learned. Dr. Peavey's study, on the other hand, employed a long-term comprehensive approach to stress management, and that might account for her differential findings. Stress as a suppressor of immune function has been well studied. It is logical that any treatment that reduces stress should help restore the integrity of the immune system.

In both the Hall study and Peavey's work, no attempt was made to control any particular type or activity of the white blood cells. Their work is extremely promising, however, because it demonstrates that, through conscious effort, the immune system can be encouraged to function in a way known to be more conducive to health. Also the studies do imply a kind of control, in that the appropriate conditions are set up for the body's own wisdom (that great superintelligence) to move in a healthy direction. Since both investigators conducted only a limited number of blood analyses, their procedures may have had a more widespread effect on the immune system than they were able to identify.

Imagery and the Neutrophil

What are the far limits of our ability to consciously communicate with body function? Twenty years ago, J. V. Basmajian, a physician and scientist, published an article in *Science* providing evidence that human beings could learn voluntary control over a single cell. When very small electrodes that could measure the electrical activity of a cell were inserted into a motor nerve cell, and auditory feedback was given to the person whenever that cell would fire, he/she could quickly learn to fire it at will. They could even learn to fire long bursts that sounded like drum rolls when they came across the speakers, or short bursts, or patterns of their own choosing.[42]

Basmajian's work; research coming from Barbara Brown and Joe Kamiya and other laboratories around the country that showed that brain waves could be similarly controlled provided feedback was given; studies of the physiology of yogis in India, who could indeed perform wondrous feats—all this defied what everyone was relatively sure was true about the human nervous system. That is, all these studies showed that functions thought to be totally beyond conscious control were quite controllable with specialized practice, and normally that appeared to require feedback of some kind. It is widely believed that no learning can occur without feedback. (How else would you know whether you'd done it right or not?) For industrialized, modernized society, that feedback has been through the medium of highly accurate machines that have been developed to measure physiology and then feed back the information in a thousand fancy ways: lights, digital readouts, bleeps, hums, and even computer graphics. Biofeedback has come into its own.

There has not been a body function that couldn't be controlled to some extent once it was adequately monitored and information provided to the subject through rapid feedback. The immune system should prove no exception. The ability to conquer all infectious and immune-related disease should come on the heels of the technology that would allow for just such monitoring. We are faced with two lags, though: First, a noninvasive technology for constantly monitoring the blood has not been developed; and second, the appropriate numbers and components of the immune system for fighting any single disease are not known.

New research suggests that monitoring and feedback may be unnecessary to communicate with the immune system, and that through the use of an imagery procedure, desired and highly specific changes can occur. We saw glimmers of this early in the biofeedback work. Barbara Brown related her surprise at discovering that her subjects could create alpha brain waves when asked to do so, without any equipment feedback, but only after they had spent some time on the brain monitoring equipment (EEG), and learned to associate a feeling state (or some kind of imagery) with the production of alpha. They simply recreated this mental state and the alpha waves were produced.[43] The yogis, too, scarcely use electronic feedback. They become attuned to their own functioning after years of quietly listening to it. Control naturally follows. We all have the capability to develop our brains in this manner, as the most exquisite biofeedback instrument of all. The time and commitment necessary to accomplish such a task, however, require an almost religious dedication. Indeed, for the yogis, physiological control is a demonstration of their spirituality.

At Michigan State University, several investigators, including C. Wayne Smith and John Schneider, have repeatedly tested the relationship between the imagination and the immune system. Their findings suggest that the imagination, in and of itself, without years and years of meditation training, and without biofeedback, can control certain functions of the neutrophils.[44]

Their first study was conducted with eight males and eight females, most of whom were students in medicine and psychology. The selected subjects were all healthy, and were carefully screened. Only those who believed they might be able to consciously control their immune system were accepted into the study. They also had to agree to attend six sessions. During the first session, bloods were drawn twice (a baseline measure), and the subjects filled out personality inventories. The second session involved a discussion of white blood cell function, and the subjects were shown slides of neutrophils, which would later be incorporated into their imagery. A relaxation and general imagery tape was played during the third session. The fourth and fifth sessions constituted training: the rationale and purpose of the study was explained, and suggestions for effective imagery were given. The group then practiced imaging and drew pictures of their imagery, which were rated according to specified criteria.

The imagery procedure involved advising the group to visualize the neutrophils changing shape, sticking to the vessel wall and passing through and then going to places where garbage had collected. The white blood cells were described as garbage collectors that picked up trash and dumped it outside the body. The procedure lasted twenty minutes. It was suggested to the subjects that they be playful with their images, and that they alter the procedure any way that seemed sensible to them. Articles clarifying the imagery studies and describing white blood cell function were sent home with them to read.

At the sixth session, blood was drawn, the relaxation and specific imagery instructions were repeated, and blood was drawn again. The images were scored by three raters who had no prior knowledge of the results of the bloodwork. The scoring system constituted another study, where numerous correlations between the bloodwork and dimensions modified from the Image CA were found.

The total white blood cell count dropped significantly from pre- to postsession (from 8200 ± 1500 to 6400 ± 1300). These results could have happened only one time in 10,000 by chance. *All* sixteen subjects showed a drop in count, and the average percentage of neutrophils that left the blood stream was 60%. More surprising, the drop in total white blood cell count was almost totally attributable to the neutrophils; the other white blood cells did not exit. The imagery was highly specific, it appears, to the neutrophils.

However, the neutrophils also showed a significant drop in adherence, or the ability to cling to the vessel walls. This initially puzzled the investigators, since the subjects had been asked to imagine an increase in adherence. They then hypothesized that it was possible that all of the responsive cells had already left the blood stream, in view of the great decrease in numbers of circulating neutrophils. So, another group of subjects was taken through an identical training procedure, only this time they were asked to image the neutrophils staying in the blood stream, and continuing to adhere. This time the adherence *increased* during the imagery procedure. The mean percentage of cells adhering after the first experiment was 28%, after the second, 56%.

The authors continue to replicate these results with tighter and tighter controls. Preliminary replications have taken place in several laboratories. The conclusions remain constant, and the effect consistent, and far exceeding any chance expectations. Imagery appears to have a direct impact on the function of the neutrophils, at least for those who believe it will.

Epilogue

After some concerted effort at using the imagination to achieve health, physical sensations and word pictures disappear, and brain waves change from semi-wide-awake alpha levels to deeper states. The imageless, wordless void is experienced as a state of unity, of divine harmony. The strife for physical health becomes irrelevant in the grand scheme; the magic remains; the spirit triumphs.

And finally, the imagination should not be regarded as a panacea for all that ails the human species—unless, of course, we choose to believe there are no limits to consciousness and its inherent ability to alter the state of things.

Appendices

Appendices

Appendix A

Imagery Script from Samuels and Bennett

"Close your eyes. Breathe in and out slowly and deeply. Relax your whole body by whatever method works best for you. Then let your ideas of all disease symptoms . . . become bubbles in your consciousness. Now imagine that these bubbles are being blown out of your mind, out of your body, out of your consciousness, by a breeze which draws them away from you, far into the distance, until you no longer see them or feel them. Watch them disappear over the horizon.

Now imagine that you are in a place that you love. It may be the beach, in the mountains, on the desert, or wherever else you feel fully alive, comfortable, and healthy. Imagine the area around you is filled with bright, clear light. Allow the light to flow into your body, making you brighter, and filling you with the energy of health. Enjoy basking in this light. . . ."[1]

Appendix B

Imagery Script Adapted From Irving Oyle

The basic instructions are as follows: (1) Find a safe place, get comfortable, close your eyes. (2) Focus thoughts on breathing; inhale and count 1000, 2000, 3000, 4000; exhale and count backwards, 4000, 3000, 2000, 1000. (3) On inhalation, imagine a wave of energy coming up the front of the body; and as you exhale, imagine the energy moving over the top of your head, down your back, and exiting at your heels. (4) Imagine a beautiful place with all of its sights, sounds, and smells; and imagine how your own body feels in such a place. Continue with the breathing exercise, allowing the energy to flow, and stay with the imaginary place in your thoughts for fifteen minutes—but keep focusing on breathing and allowing the energy to flow. (5) Look around the beautiful place for a creature; it might be an animal, a person, or even a plant. This life form is your ally, spirit guide, advisor, psychoanalyst. (6) Make friends, ask its name, continue concentrating on the breathing. Spend some time discussing the problem with this creature of the imagination, and listen for her/his advice. (7) Ask if she or he is willing to meet with you daily. (8) To seal the deal, ask the creature to give you a sign of power—either symptom relief or an answer to a problem.[2]

The instructions for what Oyle calls "Operating Your Biocomputer" are the first and most reliable medicine known to humanity—depicted on the caves that housed our ancestors during the Paleolithic period, and continued in song and totem. I would, from my own experiences, caution you never to take this exercise lightly. A slightly altered sensorium occasioned by the breathing patterns, the

levels of reality that the psyche weaves into the twilight of awareness, and the material that springs up after being embedded deeply in
the subconscious (usually for good reason), compose the ingredients
for a sometimes frightening, always emotionally charged, experience. Incidentally, you may want to do as the Indians do to test the
validity of the spirit ally. Ask it to appear to you in some form in
ordinary, everyday, wide-awake reality within the next few days.

Appendix C

Relaxation, Imagery and Pre-Biofeedback Transcript

The purpose of this tape is to learn how to relax and to decrease any pain or any anxiety you might be experiencing. Before I begin, however, I would like for you to get situated, in your chair or on your bed, in such a way that you can become totally relaxed and comfortable. Begin now by concentrating on your breathing—inhaling and exhaling—completely thinking to yourself, "relax." Inhale. Exhale. Again . . . and again. Whenever you feel tension or pain or anxiety during this tape, I would like for you to breathe deeply and say to yourself, "relax." Inhale. Exhale. Relax. If thoughts creep in while we are going through this relaxation procedure, simply encapsulate them in a bubble and let them float away.

Now, concentrating only on the sound of my voice, allowing yourself a few minutes for total relaxation, gently close your eyes and, as I count down from ten to one, think of yourself getting more and more relaxed . . . letting all of the tension and stress flow out. Relax to deeper levels than you can recall: ten, nine, eight, seven, six, five, four, three, two, one, zero. Very good.

Now, let's take a mental trip through your body so that we can identify any remaining tension or anxiety. Begin with your feet: think of them getting very heavy, relaxing, warming, sinking down. First, your right foot; then, your left foot. Become aware of each of your toes . . . they are beginning to tingle. Simply imagine all of the tension flowing out of your feet, allowing the muscles to become very loose and very smooth, tingling, warm. Now, think for a moment about your legs, your calves. Particularly your right calf: imagine any muscles that are knotted becoming smooth, warm. Your left calf. Your thighs . . . your right thigh, your left thigh . . . muscles unknotting, lengthening, warming, all the tension leaving them. Focus now on your hips, letting any tension resolve, and on your abdomen. Many of us hold a lot of stress and tightness in our abdomens. Let it dissipate, let it free. Think for a moment about your back . . . all the muscles, many, many muscles up and down your back. Let them go . . . warming, comforting. Your shoulders, let them drop slightly, letting go of any burdens. You are feeling very comfortable now. I want you to think about your right arm, the upper part of your arm, the lower part, and of your right hand. Turn them loose for a moment of any responsibilities, letting go, relaxing. Left arm, first the upper part and then the lower part, then your hand. Now in your mind's eye, travel up into the muscles of your neck. Mentally circle your neck, letting all of the tension flow out. Concentrate for a moment on your jaw. Let it drop slightly. Let it become as relaxed as possible. Focus on the right side of your face, relaxing, warming, smoothing. Then the left side of your face, relaxing, feeling very comfortable now. Now, all the muscles around your eyes, relax. All around your head, the top part of your head, the back part of your head. See the knots unwinding, the anxiety and fear and tension flowing out.

Now, give yourself a few seconds to take another mental trip through your body, identifying any tension remaining. Let it flow out. Allow yourself to achieve new levels of relaxation, of comfort. Remember that when you relax like this, your body begins to heal itself and you become energized for any activities you have ahead of you. Now, for the next few minutes, you will hear the sounds of ocean waves. Continue relaxing, allowing yourself this time to be worry-free, allowing your body to mend itself.

Appendix D

Bodymind Imagery: Taking a Mental Journey:
The Disease

Take a mental journey, now, without censoring any of the images that pop up. Some will jump into your mind with a life of their own; others will take form as you mentally sculpt them with your imagination. Focus on the area of disturbance. Softening up all around it, allow your mind to enter in. Stay soft and relaxed. Reach out now and touch whatever bothers you. Feel its texture. Smell it and take note of the odor. Listen: it's saying something. Open the eyes of your imagination. Move through your problem and around it. Remember not to be critical. Be playful, if you wish. Let the shape you've created move and change. Give it a name. Notice your feeling state.

Personal Defenses

Take a second to let these images fade. Breathe yourself into an even deeper state of relaxation. Knowing that within you lives the capacity to get well from almost anything, let that capacity take shape. It might be the immune system, or a network of highly specialized repair mechanics, or a change in structures. Watch this. Center yourself, go down into your body, until you can see and feel this happening. Create the pictures if they don't come alone. Is the defense system working? If so, how? Ask questions and listen. Let your defenses come to you in any form they wish. Remember them.

Treatment

Allow the images to fade. Now, if you are receiving any treatment, begin to imagine taking it. Observe what happens after it enters your body, where it goes. Watch its shape and color. Feel it interacting with your cells. What is it doing with them or to them? Give yourself plenty of time here. If you have more than one type of therapy, imagine the others, too. Note your emotional state as these things all interact inside. Don't be critical. Trust yourself. Trust the oldest method of diagnosis and healing known.[3]

Appendix E

Burn Imagery Transcript

I want you to get comfortable on your bed or your chair. Put all of your thoughts away . . . get comfortable and close your eyes and just relax and listen . . . relax and listen. You might even let yourself get a little sleepy. Just feel good for a little while. Close your eyes. Take a deep breath . . . let it all out. Let yourself sink back . . . feeling good . . . feeling better all the time.

As I count down from ten to one, let each count be a signal to get more and more relaxed: ten, nine, eight, seven, six, five . . . more and more comfortable now . . . four, three, two, one.

Relax your feet now, letting them get warm and comfortable. Relax your legs and let them get soothed and calm. Feeling heavier now. Relax, letting all the tension out of your stomach. Relax your hips, deeper and deeper, more and more. Take another deep breath, exhale. Let all of the tension go out. Now relax your back . . . all up and down your back. Your neck, your shoulders. Your right arm is now relaxing, and your right hand. Feeling more and more peaceful. Your left arm and your left hand are relaxed. Deeper and deeper . . . it feels good to relax . . . to get calm . . . a little more and more. Now your face, your head . . . relaxing, deeper and deeper. Your head may be feeling heavy, warm.

At the count of three, let go of any tension you may still have: one, two, three.

Feeling comfortable now, maybe a little drowsy, eyes closed. While I talk now about your treatment, just relax. And remember, whenever you feel tense or fearful, just take a deep breath and say, "relax, peace, calm." Just let the fear go.

Imagine now that the time approaches for you to get your dress-
ings taken off and go to the bath. Picture this in your imagination.
Just relax, deeper and deeper, breathing deeply whenever you feel
uncomfortable. The nurse comes in now and starts to cut your bandage off. Imagine this happening. Whenever you feel uncomfortable,
breathe, relax. Imagine this happening, feeling the nurse cut the
bandage off and your skin feeling the coolness. Take a deep breath
and let any discomfort go, feeling relaxed and calm now. As she
unwraps the bandages and takes them off, you become aware of a
feeling of coolness. Let this happen. All discomfort passes. Take
a deep breath. Let any discomfort go. Staying very relaxed and
calm now, you begin to get out of your bed . . . maybe by yourself.
You are relaxed and calm and feeling very good. Imagine yourself
moving now toward the door, moving down the hall toward your
bath . . . feeling rather cool, but no pain. Breathing deeply and
deeply, exercising your muscles with each step . . . longer and
stronger. Keep breathing. Exercise your lungs with each breath. Remember to exhale completely, relaxing.

At the count of three, I want you to let go of any tension you
might have any place in your body: one, two, three.

See yourself moving now as you approach the bath. You see the
person there who will be helping you when you need help. As you
move into the bath, you feel the water. It feels strong at first . . . and
gradually more and more comfortable. Your skin will begin to feel
good under the water . . . very clean and soothed. The burned skin
that is no longer alive needs to be rubbed off so that your new skin
can grow. When this becomes uncomfortable, remember to take a
deep breath and let the moment pass . . . staying very relaxed and
calm . . . letting the good feeling of the warm water take your
attention.

Continue to relax now, deeper and deeper, looking forward to
your return to your bed, and perhaps a nap.

You see yourself getting out of the bath now, drying off gently,
and covering yourself now as you return to your bed or your chair,
staying very calm and very relaxed. Let the discomfort pass. If you
must wait for awhile, use this time to continue to relax . . . as you
are doing now, dozing just a little. You may feel chilled, but that's
natural and will go away when your bandages are put back on. Feeling
very good now, relax more and more. Now the nurse comes in with
your new bandages. First, white soothing cream is put on your burns.
This feels very good, very soothing and smooth. As soon as it touches
your skin, it feels very good. Now, fine mesh gauze is placed over

the cream and any remaining discomfort begins to leave. New bandages are put on. You feel warmer and warmer each minute. All discomfort fades now.

Remember to work with your treatment by letting your body stay relaxed like this, feeling good, breathing deeply. Whenever you feel discomfort, inhale, exhale completely. Now, for the next few minutes, imagine yourself well, healthy, in the most beautiful place imaginable. Continue to breath deeply: inhale, and exhale, relax, relax, relax.

Rank Order of Significant Dependent Measures of Pain and Anxiety for Burn Patients

Treatments assigned the same rank order were not significantly different.

4 = Most Improved
1 = Least Improved

DEPENDENT VARIABLE	Group Control	Relaxation	Relaxation Imagery	Relaxation Imagery/ Biofeedback
Peripheral Temperature— Training	1	4	4	4
Electromyelograph— Treatment— Midsession	1	2	4	3
Subjective Units of Discomfort— Training	1	2	4	4
Subjective Units of Discomfort— Treatment	1	2	4	4
Spielberger's State Anxiety				
Post-Training	1	4	4	4
Post-Treatment	1	2	4	4
Minor Pain Medications	1	1	4	3
Sedatives	1	2	4	3

Appendix F

PURPOSEFUL ACTION

(+) POSITIVE IMAGERY
(+) HYSTERIA (MMPI)
(+) CONTROL (MMPI)
(+) ANXIETY (POMS)
(−) EXPRESSED INCLUSION (FIRO)
(−) WANTED INCLUSION (FIRO)
(−) CHANCE (L of C)

(+) RED BLOOD CELLS
(+) WHITE BLOOD CELLS
(−) HEMOGLOBIN

NON-DIRECTED STRUGGLE

(+) PSYCHASTHENIA (MMPI)
(+) F (MMPI)
(−) CHANCE (L of C)
(−) AFFECTION (FIRO)
(+) DEPRESSION (POMS)
(+) PSYCHOPATH. (MMPI)
(−) HYSTERIA (MMPI)
(+) POWERFUL OTHERS (L of C)

(+) RED BLOOD CELLS
(−) HEMOGLOBIN
(+) MEAN CORPUSCULAR VOL.
(+) MEAN CORPUSCULAR COUNT

RESIGNATION

(+) DEPRESSION (MMPI)
(+) TENSION (POMS)
(−) HYSTERIA (MMPI)
(−) SCHIZOPHRENIA (MMPI)

(+) RED BLOOD CELLS
(−) HEMOGLOBIN
(+) MCV
(+) MCC
(−) SEGS
(−) LYMPHOCYTES

Appendix G

Significant Correlations of Selected IMAGE CA and Hematology and Blood Chemistry Variables

| Variable | IMAGE CA | | | | Metaphoric Imagery | | | |
| | Cancer | | WBC | | Cancer | | | |
	AC	ST	AC	ST	CO	DA	ST	AC
Blood Meas.:								
RBC			29	32		33		30
HGB			30	27		35*		31
HCT		−30				36*	25	42*
Platelet			28			29		
WBC								25
Protein						26		
Phosphorus			−25	−32				
Uric acid			29					
Creatinine				25				
Alk. phos.	37*				35			
SGOT	26							

*p<0.01; All others significant at p<0.05.
Note:
AC = activity
ST = strength
CO = color
DA = dangerousness

Notes

Notes to Chapter 1
1. R. F. Kraus, "A Psychoanalytic Interpretation of Shamanism," pp. 19–32.
2. R. L. Bergman, "A School for Medicine Men," p. 663.
3. J. Rothenberg, *Technicians of the Sacred.*
4. W. LaBarre, "Shamanic Origins of Religion and Medicine," pp. 7–11.
5. M. Eliade, *Shamanism: Archaic Techniques of Ecstasy.*
6. Ibid.
7. L. G. Peters, and D. Price-Williams, "Towards an Experiential Analysis of Shamanism," pp. 398–418.
8. J. A. Wike, "Modern Spirit Dancing of Northern Puget Sound."
9. See note 5 above.
10. M. J. Harner, *The Way of the Shaman.*
11. G. Majno, *The Healing Hand.*
12. A. S. Lyons, and R. J. Petrucelli, *Medicine: An Illustrated History.*
13. W. B. Cannon, "Voodoo Death," pp. 182–190; S. C. Cappannari et al., "Voodoo in the General Hospital," pp. 938–940; J. R. Saphir et al., "Voodoo Poisoning in Buffalo, New York," pp. 437–438.
14. W. LaBarre, *The Peyote Cult.*
15. Harner, *Way of the Shaman,* p. xii.
16. J. Frank, *Persuasion and Healing.*
17. A. Johannes, "Many Medicines in One," pp. 43– 70.
18. R. Grossinger, *Planet Medicine,* p. 13; ibid., p. 23.
19. L. Jilek-Aall, *Call Mama Doctor.*
20. V. Garrison, "Doctor, Espiritista, or Psychiatrist?", pp. 65–180.
21. Harner, *Way of the Shaman,* p. 45.
22. Kendall, "Supernatural Traffic: East Asian Shamanism," p. 180.
23. See note 1 above.
24. Kendall, "Supernatural Traffic," p. 171.
25. S. Rogers, "Shamans and Medicine Men," pp. 1202–1223.
26. R. H. Lowie, *Primitive Religion;* D. Landy, *Culture, Disease and Healing;* M. Eliade, *Shamanism.*

27. J. Halifax, *Shamanic Voices*, p. 11.
28. A. A. Popov, "How Sereptic Djarvoskin of the Nganasans (Tavgi Samoyeds) Became a Shaman."
29. W. G. Jilek, *Indian Healing*, p. 64; ibid., p. 66; ibid.
30. Ibid., p. 73; ibid., pp. 73–74.
31. G. B. Risse, "Shamanism: The Dawn of a Healing Profession," p. 22.
32. C. Castaneda, *The Teachings of Don Juan*; idem, *A Separate Reality*.
33. A. Hultkrantz, "A Definition of Shamanism," pp. 25–37.
34. C. T. Tart, *States of Consciousness*.
35. See note 7 above.
36. E. Underhill, *Mysticism*; W. James, *The Variety of Religious Experience*.
37. L. LeShan, *The Medium, the Mystic, and the Physicist*.
38. See note 7 above.
39. LeShan, *Medium, Mystic, and Physicist*, p. 42.
40. Ibid., p. 108.
41. LeShan, *Medium, Mystic, and Physicist*; F. Capra, *The Turning Point*.
42. J. Kamiya, from material presented to the International Conference on Science and Shamanism, Esalen Institute, Big Sur, California, in February, 1984.
43. C. T. Tart, "A Psychophysiological Study of Out-of-the-Body Experiences in Selected Subjects," pp. 1–16.
44. Castaneda, *Teachings of Don Juan*.
45. P. Suedfeld, *Restricted Environmental Stimulation*.
46. W. Heron, "The Pathology of Boredom, " pp. 52–56; J. Zubek, C. Welch, and M. Saunders, "Electroencephalographic Changes During and After 14 Days of Perceptual Deprivation," pp. 490–492.
47. See note 45 above.
48. P. Suedfeld, and R. A. Borrie, "Altering States of Consciousness through Sensory Deprivation."
49. J. C. Lilly, *The Center of the Cyclone*; idem, *The Deep Self*.
50. M. Zuckerman, "Hallucinations, Reported Sensations, and Images."
51. Suedfeld, *Restricted Environmental Stimulation*, p. 44.
52. C. Wissler, *The American Indian*; E. M. Loeb, "The Shaman of Niue," pp. 393–402; P. Radin, *Primitive Religion*.
53. G. Devereux, *Basic Problems of Ethnopsychiatry*; J. Silverman, "Shamanism and Acute Schizophrenia," pp. 21–31.
54. W. G. Jilek, *Indian Healing*, p. 35.
55. R. Noll, "Shamanism and Schizophrenia," pp. 443–459.
56. See note 5 above.
57. See note 10 above.
58. Noll, "Shamanism and Schizophrenia," p. 452.
59. K. Wilber, *The Atman Project*; E. Green, and A. Green, *Beyond Biofeedback*; J. Hillman, *Re-Visioning Psychology*.
60. R. D. Laing, *The Politics of Experience*; J. W. Perry, "Reconstitutive Process in the Psychopathology of the Self," pp. 853–876.
61. I. Oyle, *Magic, Mysticism and Modern Medicine*.
62. See note 5 above.
63. Wilber, *Atman Project*, p. 152; ibid., p. 158; ibid., p. 159.
64. C. Blacker, *The Catalpa Bow*.
65. A. Lommel, *Shamanism*, p. 60.

66. M. Eliade, "Some Observations on European Witchcraft."
67. W. Y. Evans-Wentz, *Tibetan Yoga and Secret Doctrines.*
68. H. C. Guyton, *Human Physiology and Mechanisms of Disease.*
69. I will not attempt to document these common findings. The best source
    of information on scientific work in this area is the quarterly
    journal *Biofeedback and Self-Regulation.*
70. M. J. Harner, *The Way of The Shaman.*
71. O. Nordland, "Shamanism as an Experience of the 'Unreal,'" p. 174.
72. Harner, *Hallucinogens and Shamanism;* R. G. Wasson, *Divine Mushroom of
    Immortality;* W. LaBarre, *The Peyote Cult,* P. T. Furst, ed., *Flesh of
    the Gods.*
73. D. C. Noel, *Seeing Castaneda.*
74. From an interview with Sam Keen, published in Noel, *Seeing Castaneda.*
75. J. Siskind, "Visions and Cures among the Sharanahua."
76. Ibid, p. 37; ibid.
77. From Prem Das, quoted by Halifax, *Shamanic Voices,* frontispiece.
78. Ibid.
79. Wasson, *Divine Mushroom of Immortality.*
80. H. Munn, "The Mushrooms of Language."
81. Ibid., p. 88.
82. Ibid., p. 95.
83. Harner, *Hallucinogens and Shamanism;* Eliade, "European Witchcraft."
84. J. de Bergamo (c. 1470–71), "Quaestio de Strigis," p. 199.
85. See note 70 above.
86. Grossinger, *Planet Medicine,* pp. 42–43.
87. D. K. Stat, "Ancient Sound: The Whistling Vessels of Peru," pp. 2–7.
88. Bergman, "School for Medicine Men," pp. 663–666.
89. N. Drury, *The Shaman and the Magician.*
90. Resources: Tapes of shamanic drumming are available from the Center
    for Shamanic Studies, Box 673, Belden Station, Norwalk, Conn.,
    06852, and Indian chants and songs are available through Del
    Enterprise, Inc., Box 248, Mission, S. Dak., 57555. The audio
    tapes used with a headset eliminate some of the noise problems
    in doing shamanic work with unsympathetic neighbors close by.
91. Drury, *Shaman and Magician,* p. 8
92. See note 68 above.
93. R. Melzack and P. D. Wall, "Pain Mechanism: A New Theory,"
    pp. 971–979.
94. A. Neher, "Auditory Driving Observed with Scalp Electrodes in Normal
    Subjects," pp. 449–451; idem, "A Physiological Explanation of
    Unusual Behaviour in Ceremonies Involving Drums,"
    pp. 151–160.
95. Green and Green, *Beyond Biofeedback.*
96. Jilek, *Indian Healing.*
97. E. D. Adrian, and B. H. C. Matthews, "The Berger Rhythm,"
    pp. 355–385; F. Morrell, and H. H. Jasper, "Electrographic Stud-
    ies of the Formation of Temporary Connections in the Brain,"
    pp. 201–215; and many others.
98. E. R. John, and K. F. Killam, "Electrophysiological Correlates of Avoid-
    ance Conditioning in the Cat," pp. 252–274.

99. H. Benson, *The Relaxation Response;* idem, J. F. Beary, and M. P. Carol, "The Relaxation Response," pp. 37–46.
100. Benson, *Relaxation Response.*
101. Blacker, *Catalpa Bow.*
102. A. Balikci, "Shamanistic Behavior among the Netsilik Eskimos."
103. Wasson, *Divine Mushroom of Immortality.*
104. LaBarre, "Shamanic Origins."
105. M. J. Gage, *Women, Church and State*, p. 281.
106. See note 5 above.
107. S. Krippner, and A. Villoldo, *The Realms of Healing.*
108. Kraus, "Psychoanalytic Interpretation of Shamanism," p. 26.
109. Noll, "Shamanism and Schizophrenia," p. 445.
110. Rogers, "Shamans and Medicine Men."
111. T. T. Waterman, "The Paraphernalia of the Cuwamish 'Spirit-Canoe' Ceremony."
112. J. H. Tenzel, "Shamanism and Concepts of Disease in a Mayan Indian Community," pp. 372–380.
113. E. R. Service, *A Profile of Primitive Culture.*
114. W. Wildschut, "Crow Indian Medicine Bundles."
115. G. A. Reichard, *Navaho Religion.*
116. Bergman, "School for Medicine Men," p. 666.
117. Grossinger, *Planet Medicine*, p. 97.

Notes for Chapter 2
1. R. Grossinger, *Planet Medicine.*
2. A. S. Lyons, and R. J. Petrucelli, *Medicine: An Illustrated History*, p. 170.
3. From Phillimores Apollonius of Tyans, Book II, Chap. XXXVII.
4. Three excellent resources for the history of medicine during this era are: G. A. Binder, *Great Moments in Medicine;* W. Osler, *The Evolution of Modern Medicine;* Lyons and Petrucelli, *Medicine.*
5. M. J. Gage, *Women, Church and State*, p. 241.
6. Ibid., p. 242.
7. Ibid., p. 243.
8. M. Murray, *The Witch Cult in Western Europe.*
9. M. Eliade, "Some Observations on European Witchcraft," p. 41.
10. From personal communication with M. J. Harner, 1982; Harner, ed., *Hallucinogens and Shamanism.*
11. Harner, *Hallucinogens and Shamanism.*
12. M. B. Kreig, *Green Medicine: The Search for Medicines that Heal.*
13. E. Maple, *Magic, Medicine, and Quackery.*
14. Ibid., p. 43.
15. Lyons and Petrucelli, *Medicine.*
16. Quoted by Maple, *Magic, Medicine, and Quackery*, p. 67.
17. B. Ehrenreich, and D. English, *Witches, Midwives, and Nurses.*
18. Quoted by H. R. Trevor-Roper, *The European Witch-Craze of the Sixteenth and Seventeenth Centuries and Other Essays*, p. 142.
19. G. Zilboorg, *The Medicine Man and the Witch during the Renaissance*, p. 62.
20. M. Harris, *Cows, Pigs, Wars and Witches.*
21. M. Daly, *Gyn/Ecology: The Metaethics of Radical Feminism.*

22. See Gage, *Women, Church and State,* for a breakdown in expenses for burning a witch in France.
23. Quoted by F. Capra, *The Turning Point.*
24. Capra, *Turning Point,* p. 56.
25. Osler, *Modern Medicine,* p. 187.
26. A. M. Stoddart, *Life of Paracelsus,* p. 213.
27. F. Hartman, *Paracelsus: Life and Prophecies,* pp. 111–112.
28. C. E. McMahon, "The Role of Imagination in the Disease Process," p. 181.
29. F. Sommers, "Dualism in Descartes."

Notes for Chapter 3
1. N. Cousins, *The Healing Heart,* p. 16.
2. J. Achterberg, I. Collerain, and P. Craig, "A Possible Relationship between Cancer, Mental Retardation, and Mental Disorders," pp. 135–139.
3. D. Costa, E. Mestes, and A. Coban, "Breast and Other Cancer Deaths in a Mental Hospital," pp. 371–378.
4. See S. E. Locke and M. Hornig-Rohan, *Mind and Immunity,* for an annotated bibliography of this material.
5. J. W. Berg, R. Ross, and H. B. Latourette, "Economic Status and Survival of Cancer Patients." pp. 467–477.
6. J. Frank, *Persuasion and Healing.*
7. Ibid., p. 138.
8. M. Lorr, D. M. McNair, and G. H. Weinstein, "Early Effects of Librium Used with Psychotherapy," pp. 257–270.
9. F. A. Volgyesi, "School for Patients," pp. 8–17.
10. S. Wolf, "Effects of Suggestion and Conditioning on the Action of Chemical Agents in Human Subjects," pp. 100–109.
11. Cousins, *Human Options,* pp. 19–20.
12. J. Achterberg, and G. F. Lawlis, *Bridges of the Bodymind;* L. LeShan, *The Mechanic and the Gardener;* L. Dossey, *Space, Time and Medicine;* J. D. Goldstrich, *The Best Chance Diet;* D. Ornish, *Stress, Diet and Your Heart;* O. C. Simonton, S. Simonton, and J. Creighton, *Getting Well Again.*
13. J. H. Schultz, and W. Luthe, *Autogenic Training.*
14. G. Dick-Read, *Childbirth without Fear,* p. 14.
15. D. Brook, *Naturebirth,* p. 133; ibid., p. 127.
16. C. Garfield, "Beyond the Relaxation Response."
17. Brook, *Naturebirth,* p. 130.
18. From Demographic Yearbooks, statistics published by the United Nations.
19. D. Haire, and J. Haire, "The Cultural Warping of Childbirth."
20. J. E. Johnson, "Effects of Accurate Expectations about Sensations on the Sensory and Distress Components of Pain," pp. 261–275; idem et al., "Sensory Information Instruction in a Coping Strategy, and Recovering from Surgery," pp. 4–17.
21. D. Krieger, *Therapeutic Touch.*
22. Achterberg and Lawlis, *Imagery of Cancer.*

23. These materials were presented by Dr. Heidt at the Second Annual Conference on Imaging and Fantasy Process, November 1978, and case studies were published in Achterberg and Lawlis, *Bridges of the Bodymind.*
24. Achterberg and Lawlis, *Bridges of the Bodymind.*
25. M. Samuels and H. Bennett, *Be Well,* p. 144.
26. M. Samuels and N. Samuels, *Seeings with the Mind's Eye;* Samuels and Bennett, *The Well Body Book;* idem, *Be Well.*
27. I. Oyle, *Magic, Mysticism and Modern Medicine,* p. 11.
28. Ibid., p. 34.
29. Oyle, *The New American Medical Show,* p. 149.
30. J. Segal, "Biofeedback as a Medical Treatment," p. 149.
31. Several good sources on the technical aspects of biofeedback are: E. Green, and A. Green, *Beyond Biofeedback;* K. R. Gaarder, and P. Montgomery, *Clinical Biofeedback: A Procedural Manual;* B. Brown, *New Mind, New Body;* idem, *Stress and the Art of Biofeedback;* D. S. Olton, and A. R. Noonberg, *Biofeedback: Clinical Applications in Behavioral Medicine;* J. V. Basmajian, *Muscles Alive,* 3rd ed.; R. J. Gatchel, and K. P. Price, eds., *Clinical Applications of Biofeedback.*
32. Achterberg, P. McGraw, and Lawlis, "Rheumatoid Arthritis: A Study of Relaxation and Temperature Biofeedback as an Adjunctive Therapy," pp. 207–223.
33. The research, application and scientific references for several specific disorders were published in depth in Achterberg and Lawlis, *Bridges of the Bodymind.*
34. Statistical diagnostic procedures are available in Achterberg and Lawlis, *Imagery and Disease,* which contains work formerly published in *Imagery of Cancer* as well as evaluation tools for diabetes and spinal pain (Institute for Personality and Ability Testing, 1984). A brief discussion of the development of the cancer instrument is discussed later in Chapter 6.
35. E. Kiester, "The Playing Fields of the Mind," p. 20.
36. Achterberg, C. Kenner, and Lawlis, "Biofeedback, Imagery, and Relaxation"; Kenner and Achterberg, "Non-Pharmacologic Pain Relief for Patients."

Notes for Chapter 4
1. M. S. Gazzaniga, and J. E. Ledoux, The Integrated Mind.
2. A. Luria, *The Mind of a Mnemonist.*
3. T. X. Barber, H. H. Chauncey, and R. A. Winer, "Effects of Hypnotic and Nonhypnotic Suggestion on Paratid Gland Response to Gustatory Stimuli," pp. 374–380; K. D. White, "Salivation: The Significance of Imagery in its Voluntary Control," pp. 196–203.
4. A. E. Kazdin, and L. A. Wilcoxin, "Systematic Desensitization and Nonspecific Treatment Effects," p. 5; E. L. Digiusto, and N. Bond, "Imagery and the Autonomic Nervous System," pp. 427–438.
5. K. L. Lichstein, and E. Lipshitz, "Psychophysiological Effects of Noxious Imagery," pp. 339–345.

6. W. A. Shaw, "The Relaxation of Muscular Action Potentials to Imaginal Weight Lifting," pp. 247–250.
7. Barber, "Psychological Aspects of Hypnosis," pp. 390–419; idem, *Hypnosis: A Scientific Approach*; idem, "Hypnosis, Suggestions and Psychosomatic Phenomena," pp. 13–27.
8. J. Schneider, C. W. Smith, and S. Whitcher, "The Relationship of Mental Imagery to White Blood Cell (Neutrophil) Function"; H. R. Hall, "Hypnosis and the Immune System," pp. 92–103.
9. Kazdin and Wilcoxin, "Systematic Desensitization."
10. C. S. Jordan, and K. T. Lenington, "Physiological Correlates of Eidetic Imagery and Induced Anxiety," pp. 31–42.
11. G. E. Schwartz, D. A. Weinberger, and J. A. Singer, "Cardiovascular Differentiation of Happiness, Sadness, Anger, and Fear: Imagery and Exercise," pp. 343–364.
12. R. W. Sperry, and M. S. Gazzaniga, "Language following Surgical Disconnection of the Hemispheres," pp. 108–121; J. E. Bogen, "The Other Side of the Brain," pp. 135–162.
13. Gazzaniga and LeDoux, *Integrated Mind*; Bogen, "Other Side of the Brain"; J. Levy, C. Trevarthen, and R. W. Sperry, "Perception of Bilateral Chimeric Figures following Hemispheric Deconnection," pp. 61–78.
14. D. Galin, and R. Ornstein, "Individual Differences in Cognitive Style," pp. 367–376.
15. M. A. Safer, and H. Leventhal, "Ear Differences in Evaluating Emotional Tones of Voice and Verbal Content," pp. 75–82; D. M. Tucker et al., "Right Hemisphere Activation during Stress," pp. 697–700.
16. B. Lyman, S. Bernardin, and S. Thomas, "Frequency of Imagery in Emotional Experience," pp. 1159–1162.
17. P. Bakan, "Imagery, Raw and Cooked"; J. Head, *Aphasia and Kindred Disorders of Speech*, Vol. 1.
18. I. M. Lesser, "A Review of the Alexithymia Concept," pp. 531–543.
19. W. J. H. Nauta, "Some Efferent Connections of the Prefrontal Cortex in the Monkey."
20. C. F. Jacobsen, "Studies of Cerebral Function in Primates," pp. 3–60.
21. A. Meyer, and E. Beck, *Prefrontal Leucotomy and Related Operations.*
22. B. Milner, "Interhemispheric Differences in the Localization of Psychological Process in Man," pp. 272–277.
23. M. E. Humphrey, and O. L. Zangwill, "Cessation of Dreaming after Brain Injury," pp. 322–325.
24. M. Critchley, *The Parietal Lobes.*
25. B. Milner, "Brain Mechanisms Suggested by Studies of Temporal Lobes"; E. DeRenzi, "Nonverbal Memory and Hemispheric Side of the Lesion," pp. 181–189.
26. J. H. Jackson, "On Right or Left-Sided Spasm at the Onset of Epileptic Paroxysms, and on Crude Sensation Warnings and Elaborate Mental States," pp. 192–206.
27. W. Penfield, and P. Perot, "The Brain's Record of Auditory and Visual Experience," pp. 595–596.
28. H. Selye, *The Stress of Life.*
29. W. Herbert, "Elaborating the Stress Response."

30. A. Samuels, "Beyond the Relaxation Response."
31. H. F. Dvorak et al., "Fibrin Gel Investment Associated with Line 1 and Line 10 Solid Tumor Growth, Angiogenesis, and Fibroplasia in Guinea Pigs," pp. 1458–1472.
32. K. Lashley, "In Search of the Engram," pp. 425–482.
33. P. J. van Heerden, *The Foundation of Empirical Knowledge.*
34. K. Pribram, *Languages of the Brain;* idem, "Problems Concerning the Structure of Consciousness"; K. Wilber, *The Holographic Paradigm and Other Paradoxes;* M. Ferguson, *Karl Pribram's Changing Reality.*
35. Pribram, *Languages of the Brain,* p. 157.
36. Pribram, "What the Fuss is All About," p. 32.
37. Pribram, *Languages of the Brain,* p. 152.
38. Ibid., p. 100.
39. A. Ahsen, "Neural Experimental Growth Potential for the Treatment of Accident Traumas, Debilitating Stress Conditions, and Chronic Emotional Blocking," pp. 1–22.
40. S. Weisburd, "Food for Mind and Mood," pp. 216–219.
41. J. Achterberg et al., "Psychological Factors and Blood Chemistries as Disease Outcome Predictors for Cancer Patients," pp. 107–122; R. L. Trestman, "Imagery, Coping, and Physiological Variables in Adult Cancer Patients."
42. H. Benson, *The Relaxation Response.*
43. See D. D. Barchas et al., "Behavioral Neurochemistry," pp. 964–973, for an excellent review on behavioral neurochemistry, which emphasizes the endorphins as neuroregulators.
44. M. W. Adler, "Endorphins, Enkephalins, and Neurotransmitters," pp. 71–74.
45. J. D. Levine, N. C. Gordon, and H. L. Fields, "The Mechanism of Placebo Analgesia," pp. 654–657.
46. L. C. Saland et al., "Acute Injections of Opiate Peptides into the Rat Cerebral Ventrical," pp. 523–528.
47. S. C. Gilman et al., "Beta-Endorphin Enhances Lymphocyte Proliferative Responses," pp. 4226–4230.
48. E. Hazum, K. J. Chang, and P. Cuartrecasas, "Specific Monoplate Receptors for Beta-Endorphin," pp. 1033–1035.
49. E. W. D. Colt, W. Wardlaw, and A. G. Frantz, "The Effect of Running on Plasma Beta-Endorphin," p. 1637.
50. A. Goldstein, "Thrills in Response to Music and Other Stimuli," pp. 126–129.
51. S. Steinberg, "Endorphins: New Types and Sweet Links," p. 136.

Notes for Chapter 5
1. A. Kleinman and L. H. Sung, "Why Do Indigenous Practitioners Successfully Heal?", pp. 7–26.
2. Ibid.
3. Kleinman, "Some Issues for a Comparative Study of Medical Healing."
4. Kleinman and Sung, "Indigenous Practitioners," p. 8.
5. E. Benedict, and T. Porter, "Native Indian Medicine Ways," p. 7.
6. Z. J. Lipowski, "Psychosomatic Medicine in the Seventies," pp. 233–238.
7. Quoted by ibid., p. 233.

8. K. Pelletier, *Mind as Healer, Mind as Slayer.*
9. J. L. Singer, and K. S. Pope, eds., *The Power of the Human Imagination;*
   A. Sheikh, *Imagery: Current Theory, Research and Application;* J. E.
   Shorr et al., eds., *Imagery: Its Many Dimensions and Applications.*
10. A. Sheikh, and C. S. Jordan, "Clinical Uses of Mental Imagery."
11. Ibid., p. 423.
12. K. D. Strosahl, and J. C. Ascough, "Clinical Uses of Mental Imagery,"
    pp. 422–438.
13. D. Meichenbaum, *Cognitive-Behavioral Modification.*
14. Meichenbaum, "Why Does Using Imagery in Psychotherapy Lead to
    Change?"
15. Singer, *Imagery and Daydream Methods in Psychotherapy and Behavior
    Modification.*
16. C. Philips, and M. Hunter, "The Treatment of Tension Headache,"
    pp. 499–507; N. Spanos, C. Horton, and J. Chaves, "The Effects
    of Two Cognitive Strategies on Pain Threshold," pp. 677–681;
    J. J. Horan, F. C. Layne, and C. H. Pursell, "Preliminary Studies
    of 'In Vivo' Emotive Imagery on Dental Discomfort,"
    pp. 105–106.
17. F. H. Kanfer, "The Many Faces of Self-Control."
18. M. D. Avia, and F. H. Kanfer, "Coping with Aversive Stimulation,"
    pp. 73–81; E. L. Worthington, Jr., "The Effects of Imagery Con-
    tent, Choice of Imagery Content, and Self-Verbalization on the
    Self-Control of Pain," pp. 225–240.
19. Kleinman and Sung, "Indigenous Practitioners," p. 7.
20. E. F. Torrey, "What Western Psychotherapists Can Learn from Witch-
    doctors," pp. 69–76.
21. J. Frank, Persuasion and Healing; Kleinman and Sung, "Indigenous Prac-
    titioners," pp. 7–26.
22. R. C. Ness, and R. M. Wintrob, "Folk Healing."
23. L. D. Weatherhead, *Psychology, Religion and Healing.*
24. Frank, *Persuasion and Healing.*
25. See note 20 above.
26. G. B. Risse, "Shamanism: The Dawn of a Healing Profession," pp. 18–23.
27. J. Maddox, *The Medicine Man,* quoted by Torrey, "What Western Psychia-
    trists Can Learn," p. 73.
28. M. E. P. Seligman, *Helplessness;* W. B. Cannon, "Voodoo Death,"
    pp. 182–190.
29. Frank, *Persuasion and Healing,* p. 66.
30. Risse, "Shamanism," p. 22; ibid.
31. J. Deese, and S. H. Hulse, *The Psychology of Learning.*
32. Ness and Wintrob, "Folk Healing."
33. W. G. Jilek, *Indian Healing.*
34. R. L. Bergman, "A School for Medicine Men," pp. 663–666.

Notes for Chapter 6

1. C. Bernard, *An Introduction to the Study of Experimental Medicine,* originally
   published in 1865, revised and translated in 1957, p. 73.
2. J. Page, *Blood: The River of Life.*
3. R. Ader, ed., *Psychoneuroimmunology.*

4. R. Ader, and N. Cohen, "Behaviorally Conditioned Immunosupression and Murine Systemic Lupus Erythematosus," pp. 127–128.
5. S. E. Locke, and M. Horning-Rohan, *Mind and Immunity*.
6. M. P. Rogers, D. Dubey, and P. Reich, "The Influence of the Psyche and the Brain on Immunity and Disease Susceptibility," pp. 147–165; M. Stein, R. Schiavi, and M. Camerino, "Influence of Brain and Behavior on the Immune System," pp. 435–440.
7. E. Harrell, P. Lambert, and J. Achterberg, "The Effects of Electrical Stimulation of the Hypothalamus on Macrophagic Activity in the Rat," pp. 193–196.
8. K. Bulloch, and R. Y. Moore, "Innervation of the Thymus Gland by Brainstem and Spinal Cord in Mouse and Rat," pp. 157–166.
9. P. Bardos et al., "Neocortical Lateralization of NK Activity in Mice," pp. 609–611.
10. N. Geschwind, and P. Behan, "Left-Handedness: Association with Immune Disease, Migraine, and Developmental Learning Disorder," pp. 5097–5100.
11. Bibliography sponsored by the Reynolds Foundation and circulated in mimeograph, 1976.
12. E. Green, and A. Green, *Beyond Biofeedback*.
13. B. Klopfer, "Psychological Variables in Human Cancer," p. 334.
14. Ibid, p. 339.
15. L. LeShan, *The Mechanic and the Gardener*, p. 139.
16. Ibid.
17. A. Carrel, *Man the Unknown*.
18. Ibid., p. 314.
19. H. Selye, *The Stress of Life*.
20. S. C. Gilman et al., "Beta-Endorphin Enhances Lymphocyte Proliferative Responses," pp. 4226–4230.
21. Work conducted by investigators Plotnikoff, Miller, and Murgo at the Oral Roberts School of Medicine at Tulsa, Okla., and reported in *Science News*, Vol. 122, July 24, 1982.
22. J. Wyblan et al., "Suggestive Evidence for Receptors for Morphine and Methionine-Enkephalin on Normal Human Blood T-Lymphocytes," pp. 1068–1070.
23. H. Newman, "Health Attitudes, Locus of Control and Religious Orientation."
24. D. Gregg, "The Paucity of Arthritis among Psychotic Patients," pp. 853–854; T. L. Pilkington, "The Coincidence of Rheumatoid Arthritis and Schizophrenia," pp. 604–607.
25. Achterberg, I. Collerain, and P. Craig, "A Possible Relationship between Cancer, Mental Retardation, and Mental Disorders," pp. 135–139.
26. A. Leaf, "Every Day is a Gift When You Are over 100," pp. 93–118; S. Benet, *Abkhasians*; G. Halsel, *Los Viegos*.
27. Leaf, "Every Day is a Gift."
28. Achterberg, O. C. Simonton, and S. Simonton, "Psychology of the Exceptional Cancer Patient," pp. 416–422.
29. R. Derogatis, M. D. Abeloff, and N. Melisaratos, "Psychological Coping

Mechanisms and Survival Time in Metastatic Breast Cancer," pp. 1504–1508.

30. This work and the following studies are found in the following publications: Achterberg, et al., "Psychological Factors and Blood Chemistries as Disease Outcome Predictors for Cancer Patients," pp. 107–122; Achterberg, and G. F. Lawlis, "A Canonical Analysis of Blood Chemistry Variables Related to Psychological Measures of Cancer Patients," pp. 1–10.

31. R. L. Trestman, "Imagery, Coping, and Physiological Variables in Adult Cancer Patients."

32. This work appeared in Achterberg and Lawlis, *Imagery of Cancer: A Diagnostic Tool for the Process of Disease*, published by IPAT in 1978, and revised in 1984 to include tools for diabetes and pain under the new title *Imagery and Disease.*

33. P. Bakan, "Imagery, Raw and Cooked."

34. Detailed results on the findings of the Cancer Rehabilitation Clinic are reported in: Final Report, Cancer Rehabilitation Demonstration Project, NCI#N01-CN-45133, National Cancer Institute, National Institute of Health, Washington, D.C., 1977. The results of the laryngectomee study are reported in Final Report, Comprehensive Rehabilitation of the Laryngectomee, NCI#R18-CA-18629, National Cancer Institute, National Institute of Health, Washington, D.C., 1979.

35. M. J. Harner, personal communication.

36. L. Thomas, "On Warts."

37. Ibid., p. 62.

38. Ibid., pp. 63–64; ibid., p. 65.

39. H. R. Hall, "Hypnosis and the Immune System: A Review with Implications for Cancer and the Psychology of Healing," pp. 92–103; idem, S. Longo, and R. Dixon, "Hypnosis and the Immune System: The Effect of Hypnosis on T and B Cell Function."

40. B. S. Peavey, "Biofeedback Assisted Relaxation: Effects on Phagocytic Immune Function."

41. C. W. Smith et al., "Imagery and Neutrophil Function Studies."

42. J. V. Basmajian, "Control of Individual Motor Units," pp. 440–441.

43. B. Brown, *New Mind, New Body.*

44. J. Schneider, C. W. Smith, and S. Whitcher, "The Relationship of Mental Imagery to White Blood Cell (Neutrophil) Function."

Notes to Appendixes

1. M. Samuels, and H. Bennett, *Be Well*, p. 284.

2. I. Oyle, The New American Medical Show.

3. Over the years of conducting research projects, special scripts have been developed that serve the subtle purpose of health education. These scripts inform the patient on the nature of the disorder, and on potential sources of recovery—particularly the patient's own self-curative resources. These are on audio tape and available for diabetes, rheumatoid arthritis, pain, cancer, burn injury,

migraine, and obesity. A general relaxation tape is also available that serves as a pre-imagery, pre-biofeedback induction. Tapes are $13.50, plus $2.00 postage and handling (Texas residents add 5% sales tax), from Health Associates, Inc. P. O. Box 36471, Dallas, Tx. 75235.

Bibliography

Achterberg, J.; Collerain, I.; and Craig, P. "A Possible Relationship Between Cancer, Mental Retardation, and Mental Disorders." *Journal of Social Science and Medicine* 12 (May 1978): 135–139.

————; Kenner, C.; and Lawlis, G. F. "Biofeedback, Imagery, and Relaxation: Pain and Stress Intervention for Severely Burned Patients." Paper presented at the Biofeedback Society of America, Annual Meetings, Chicago, Ill., March, 1982.

————, and Lawlis, G. F. *Imagery of Cancer: A Diagnostic Tool for the Process of Disease.* Champaign, Ill.: Institute for Personality and Ability Testing, 1978.

————, and ————. "A Canonical Analysis of Blood Chemistry Variables Related to Psychological Measures of Cancer Patients." *Multivariate Experimental Clinical Research.* 1 & 2 vol. 4 (1979): 1–10.

————, and ————. *Bridges of the Bodymind: Behavioral Approaches to Health Care.* Champaign, Ill.: Institute for Personality and Ability Testing, 1980.

————, and ————. "Imagery and Terminal Care: The Therapist as Shaman." In *Behavior Therapy in Terminal Care,* edited by D. Sobel. Cambridge, Mass.: Ballinger, 1981.

————, and ————. *Imagery and Disease.* Champaign, Ill.: Institute for Personality and Ability Testing, 1984.

————; ————; Simonton, O. C.; and Simonton, S. "Psychological Factors and Blood Chemistries as Disease Outcome Predictors for Cancer Patients." *Multivariate Experimental Clinical Research* 3 (1977): 107–122.

————; McGraw, P.; and Lawlis, G. F. "Rheumatoid Arthritis: A Study of Relaxation and Temperature Biofeedback as an Adjunctive Therapy." *Biofeedback and Self-Regulation* 6 (1981): 207–223.

————; Simonton, O. C.; and Simonton, S. "Psychology of the Exceptional Cancer Patient: A Description of Patients Who Outlive Predicted Life Expectancies." *Psychotherapy: Theory, Research, and Practice* 14 (Winter 1977): 416–422.

Ader, R. ed. *Psychoneuroimmunology.* New York: Academia Press, 1981.

————, and Cohen, N. "Behaviorally Conditioned Immuno-supression and Murine Systemic Lupus Erythematosus." *Psychosomatic Medicine* 44 (1982): 127–128.

Adler, M. W. "Endorphins, Enkephalins, and Neurotransmitters." *Surgical Rounds,* June 1983, pp. 71–74.

Adrian, E. D. and Matthews, B. H. C. "The Berger Rhythm, Potential Changes from the Occiptal Lobes in Man." *Brain* 57 (1934): 355–385.

Ahsen, A. *Basic Concepts in Eidetic Psychotherapy.* New York: Brandon House, 1968.

————. "Eidetics: Neural Experimental Growth Potential for the Treatment of Accident Traumas, Debilitating Stress Conditions, and Chronic Emotional Blocking." *Journal of Mental Imagery* 2 (1978): 1–22.

Anderson, M. P. "Imaginal process: Therapeutic applications and theoretical models." In *Psychotherapy Process: Current Issues and Future Trends,* edited by M. J. Mahoney. New York: Plenum, 1980.

Aristotle. *Parva Naturalia.* Oxford ed., vol. III, 463a.

Assagioli, R. *Psychosynthesis: A Collection of Basic Writings.* New York: Viking, 1965.

Avia, M. D., and Kanfer, F. H. "Coping with Aversive Stimulation: The Effects of Training in a Self-Management Contest." *Cognitive Therapy and Research* 4 (1980): 73–81.

Bakan, P. "Imagery, Raw and Cooked: A Hemispheric Recipe." In *Imagery,* edited by J. E. Shorr; G. E. Sobel; P. Robin; and J. A. Connella. New York: Plenum Press, 1980.

Balikci, A. "Shamanistic Behavior among the Netsilik Eskimos." In *Magic, Witchcraft and Curing,* edited by J. Middleton. New York: The Natural History Press, 1967.

Barber, T. X. "Psychological Aspects of Hypnosis." *Psychological Bulletin* 58 (1961): 390–419.

————. *Hypnosis: A Scientific Approach.* New York: Van Nostrand, 1969.

————. "Hypnosis, Suggestions and Psychosomatic Phenomena: A New Look from the Standpoint of Recent Experimental Studies." *The American Journal of Clinical Hypnosis* 21 (1978): 13–27.

————; Chauncey, H. H.; and Winer, R. A. "Effects of Hypnotic and Nonhypnotic Suggestions on Paratid Gland Response to Gustatory Stimuli." *Psychosomatic Medicine* 26 (1964): 374–380.

Barchas, D. D.; Akil, H.; Elliott, G. R.; Holman, R. B.; and Watson, S. J. "Behavioral Neurochemistry: Neuroregulators and Behavioral States." *Science* 200 (1978): 964–973.

Bardos, P.; Degenne, D.; Lebranchu, Y.; Biziere, K.; and Renoux, G. "Neocortical Lateralization of NK Activity in Mice." *Scandinavian Journal of Immunology* 13 (1981): 609–611.

Bartrop, R. W.; Luckhurst, E.; Lazurus, L.; Kiloh, L. G.; and Penny, R. "Depressed Lymphocyte Function after Bereavement." *Lancet* 1 (1977): 834–836.

Basmajian, J. V. "Control of Individual Motor Units." *Science* 141 (1963): 440–441.

————. *Muscles Alive: Their Functions Revealed by Electromyography,* 3rd ed. Baltimore: Williams & Wilkins, 1979.

Beck, A. R. "Role of Fantasies in Psychotherapy and Psychopathology." *Journal of Nervous and Mental Diseases* 150 (1970): 3–17.

Benedict, E., and Porter, T. "Native Indian Medicine Ways." *Monchanin Journal* 10 (1977): 11–22.

Benet, S. *Abkhasians*. New York: Holt, Rinehart and Winston, 1974.

Benson, H. *The Relaxation Response*. New York: Morrow, 1975.

————: Beary, J. F.; and Carol, M. P. "The Relaxation Response." *Psychiatry* 37 (1974): 37–46.

Berg, J. W.; Ross, R.; and Latourette, H. B. "Economic Status and Survival of Cancer Patients." *Cancer* 39 (1977): 467–477.

Bergamo, J. de. (c. 1470–1471.) "Quaestio de Strigis." Unpublished manuscript, Bibliotheque National, Paris. Quoted in Joseph Hanse, *Quellen and Untersuchen zur Geschichte des Hexenwahns und der Hexenverfulgung in Mittelalter*. pp. 195–200. Bonn: Carl Georgi, 1901 (1905).

Bergman, R. L. "A School for Medicine Men." *American Journal of Psychiatry* 130, 6 (June 1973): 663–666.

Bernard, C. *An Introduction to the Study of Experimental Medicine*. New York: Dover Publications, Inc., 1957.

Binder, G. A. *Great Moments in Medicine*. Detroit: Parke-Davis, 1966.

Binet, A. *L'Etude Experimentale de l'Intelligence*. Paris: Costes, 1922.

Blacker, C. *The Catalpa Bow*. London: Allen & Unwin, 1975.

Bogen, J. E. "The Other Side of the Brain: An Oppositional Mind." *Bulletin of the Los Angeles Neurological Society* 34 (1969): 135–162.

Brook, D. *Naturebirth*. New York: Pantheon Books, 1976.

Brown, B. *New Mind, New Body*. New York: Harper & Row, 1974.

————. *Stress and the Art of Biofeedback*. New York: Harper & Row, 1977.

Bulloch, K., and Moore, R. Y. "Innervation of the Thymus Gland by Brainstem and Spinal Cord in Mouse and Rat." *American Journal of Anatomy* 161 (1981): 157–166.

Cannon, W. B. "Voodoo Death." *Psychosomatic Medicine* 19 (1957): 182–190.

Cappannari, S. C.; Rau, B.; Abram, H. S. et al. "Voodoo in the General Hospital: A Case of Hexing and Regional Enteritis." *Journal of the American Medical Association* 232 (1975): 938–940.

Capra, F. *The Turning Point*. New York: Simon & Schuster, 1982.

Carrel, A. *Man the Unknown*. New York: Harper & Row, 1935.

Castaneda, C. *The Teachings of Don Juan: A Yaqui Way of Knowledge*. Berkeley and Los Angeles: University of California Press, 1968.

————. *A Separate Reality: Further Conversations with Don Juan*. New York: Simon & Schuster, 1971.

Cautela, J. R. "Covert Conditioning: Assumptions and Procedures." *Journal of Mental Imagery* 1 (1977): 53–64.

Clark, P. "The Phantasy Method of Analyzing Narcissistic Neurosis." *Psychoanalytic Review* 13 (1925): 225–232.

Colt, E. W. D.; Wardlaw, W.; and Frantz, A. G. "The Effect of Running on Plasma Beta-Endorphin." *Life Science* 28 (1981): 1637.

Costa, D.; Mestes, E.; and Coban, A. "Breast and Other Cancer Deaths in a Mental Hospital," *Neoplasma* 28 (1981): 371–378.

Cousins, N. *Human Options*. New York: W. W. Norton & Co., 1981.

————. *The Healing Heart*. New York: W. W. Norton & Co., 1983.

Crampton, M. *An Historical Survey of Mental Imagery Techniques in Psychotherapy and Description of the Dialogic Imaginal Integration Method*. Montreal: Quebec Center for Psychosynthesis, 1974.

Critchley, M. *The Parietal Lobes*. London: Edward Arnold, 1953.

Daly, M. *Gyn/Ecology: The Metaethics of Radical Feminism*. Boston: Beacon Press, 1978.

Deese, J., and Hulse, S. H. *The Psychology of Learning*. New York: McGraw Hill, 1967.

DeRenzi, E. "Nonverbal Memory and Hemispheric Side of the Lesion." *Neuropsychologia* 6 (1968): 181–189.

Derogatis, R.; Abeloff, M. D.; and Melisaratos, N. "Psychological Coping Mechanisms and Survival Time in Metastatic Breast Cancer." *Journal of the American Medical Association* 242 (Oct. 5, 1979): 1504–1508.

DeSoille, R. *The Directed Daydream*. New York: Psychosynthesis Research Foundation, 1965.

Devereux, G. *Basic Problems of Ethnopsychiatry*. Chicago: University of Chicago Press, 1980.

Dick-Read, G. *Childbirth without Fear*. New York: Harper & Row, 1953.

DiGuisto, E. L., and Bond, N. "Imagery and the Autonomic Nervous System: Some Methodological Issues." *Perceptual and Motor Skills* 48 (1979): 427–438.

Dossey, L. *Space, Time and Medicine*. Boulder, Co: Shambhala, 1982.

Drury, N. *The Shaman and the Magician*. London, Boston, and Henley: Routledge & Kegan Paul, 1982.

Dvorak, H. F.; Dvorak, A. M.; Manseau, B. J.; Wiberg, L.; and Churchill, W. H. "Fibrin Gel Investment Associated with Line 1 and Line 10 Solid Tumor Growth, Angiogenesis, and Fibroplasia in Guinea Pigs: Role of Cellular Immunity, Myofibroblasts, Microvascular Damage, and Infarction in Line 1 Tumor Regression." *Journal of the National Cancer Institute* 62 (1978): 1458–1472.

Ehrenreich, B., and English, D. *Witches, Midwives, and Nurses: A History of Women Healers*. New York: The Feminist Press, 1973.

Eliade, M. *Shamanism: Archaic Techniques of Ecstasy*. New York: Pantheon Books, Bollingen Foundation, 1964. (Revised from original French version, 1951).

————. "Some Observations on European Witchcraft." *Occultism, Witchcraft, and Cultural Fashions*. Chicago: Chicago University Press, 1976.

Ellis, A. *Rational-Emotive Therapy and Cognitive Behavior Therapy*. New York: Springer, 1981.

Evans-Wentz, W. Y. *Tibetan Yoga and Secret Doctrines*. London: Oxford University Press, 1967.

Ferguson, M. "Karl Pribram's Changing Reality." *Re-Vision*, 1(3/4)(1978): 8–13.

Ferguson, W. K., and Bruun, G. *A Survey of European Civilization.* Boston: Houghton Mifflin Co., 1958.

Frank, J. *Persuasion and Healing.* Baltimore and London: Johns Hopkins University Press, 1974.

Frank, L. *Die Psychoanalyse.* Munich: E. Reinhardt, 1910.

Fretingny, R., and Virel, A. *L'Imagerie Mentale.* Geneva: Mont Blanc, 1968.

Furst, P. T., ed. *Flesh of the Gods: The Ritual Use of Hallucinogens.* New York: Doubleday/Natural History Press, 1972.

Gaarder, K. R., and Montgomery, P. *Clinical Biofeedback: A Procedural Manual,* 2nd ed. Baltimore: Williams & Wilkins, 1982.

Gage, M. J. *Women, Church and State.* Published in Chicago, Ill., 1893.

Galin, D., and Ornstein, R. "Individual Differences in Cognitive Style—I: Reflective Eye Movements." *Neuropsychologia* 12 (1974): 367–376.

——, and ——. "Lateral Specialization of Cognitive Modes: An EEG Study." *Psychophysiology* 9 (1976): 412–418.

Garfield, C. "Beyond the Relaxation Response." Material presented at the University of California at Los Angeles, February, 1983.

Garrison, V. "Doctor, Espiritista, or Psychiatrist? Health-Seeking Behavior in a Puerto Rican Neighborhood of New York City." *Medical Anthropology* 1 (1977): 65–180.

Gatchel, R. J., and Price, K. P., eds. *Clinical Applications of Biofeedback: Appraisal and Status.* New York: Pergamon, 1979.

Gazzaniga, M. S., and LeDoux, J. E. *The Integrated Mind.* New York: Plenum Press, 1978.

Gendlin, E. T. *Focusing.* New York: Everest House, 1978.

Gerrard, D. Preface to *Seeing with the Mind's Eye,* by M. Samuels and N. Samuels. New York: Random House, 1975.

Geschwind, N., and Behan, P. "Left-Handedness: Association with Immune Disease, Migraine, and Developmental Learning Disorder." *Proceedings of the National Academy of Sciences* 79 (1982): 5097–5100.

Gillin, J. "Magical Fright." *Psychiatry* 11 (1948): 387–400.

Gilman, S. C.; Schwartz, J. M.; Milner, R. J.; Bloom, F. E.; and Feldman, J. D. "Beta-Endorphin Enhances Lymphocyte Proliferative Responses." *Proceedings of the National Academy of Science* 79 (July 1982): 4226–4230.

Goldstein, A. "Thrills in Response to Music and Other Stimuli." *Physiological Psychology* 8 (1980): 126–129.

Goldstritch, J. D. *The Best Chance Diet.* Atlanta: Humanics Limited, 1982.

Green, E., and Green, A. *Beyond Biofeedback.* New York: Delta, 1977.

Gregg, D. "The Paucity of Arthritis Among Psychotic Patients." *American Journal of Psychiatry* (1939): 853–854.

Grossinger, R. *Planet Medicine: From Stone Age Shamanism to Post-Industrial Healing.* Garden City, New York: Anchor Press/Doubleday, 1980.

Guillerey, M. "Medicine Psychologique." In *Medecine Officielle et Medecine Heretique*. Paris: Plon, 1945.

Guyton, H. C. *Human Physiology and Mechanisms of Disease*. 3rd ed. Philadelphia: W. B. Saunders Co., 1982.

Haire, D., and Haire, J. "The Cultural Warping of Childbirth." *Special News Report*. International Childbirth Education Association, 1972.

Halifax, J. *Shamanic Voices: A Survey of Visionary Narratives*. New York: E. P. Dutton, 1979.

Hall, H. R. "Hypnosis and the Immune System: A Review with Implications for Cancer and the Psychology of Healing." *Journal of Clinical Hypnosis* 25, 2–3 (1982–1983): 92–103.

————.; Longo, S.; and Dixon, R. "Hypnosis and the Immune System: The Effect of Hypnosis on T and B Cell Function." Paper presented to the Society for Clinical and Experimental Hypnosis, 33rd Annual Workshops and Scientific Meeting, Portland, Oregon, October, 1981.

Halsel, G. *Los Viegos*. Emmaus: Rodale Press, 1976.

Happich, C. "Das Bildbewusstsein als Ansatzstelle Psychischer Behandling." Zbl. *Psychotherapie* 5 (1932): 663–667.

Harner, M. J., ed. *Hallucinogens and Shamanism*. New York: Oxford University Press, 1973.

————. *The Way of the Shaman: A Guide to Power and Healing*. San Francisco: Harper & Row, 1980.

Harrell, E.; Lambert, P.; and Achterberg, J. "The Effects of Electrical Stimulation of the Hypothalamus on Macrophagic Activity in the Rat." *Physiological Psychology*, 9, 2 (1979): 193–196.

Harris, M. *Cows, Pigs, Wars and Witches: The Riddles of Culture*. New York: Vintage Books, 1978.

Hartman, F. *Paracelsus: Life and Prophecies*. Blauvelt, N. Y.: Rudolf Steiner, 1973.

Hazum, E.; Chang, K. J.; and Cuartrecasas, P. "Specific Monoplate Receptors for Beta-Endorphins." *Science* 205 (1979): 1033–1035.

Head, J. *Aphasia and Kindred Disorders of Speech*, vol. 1. Cambridge: Cambridge University Press, 1926.

Heidt, P. "Patients Tell Their Stories." Paper presented to the second Annual Conference on Imaging and Fantasy Process, New York, 1978.

Herbert, W. "Elaborating the Stress Response." *Science News* 24 (1983): 84.

Heron, W. "The Pathology of Boredom." *Scientific American* 196 (1957): 52056.

Hillman, J. *Re-Visioning Psychology*. New York: Harper & Row, 1975.

Horan, J. J.; Layne, F. C.; and Pursell, C. H. "Preliminary Studies of in Vivo' Emotive Imagery on Dental Discomfort." *Perceptual and Motor Skills* 42 (1976): 105–106.

Horowitz, M. J. "Visual Thought Images in Psychotherapy." *American Journal of Psychotherapy* 12 (1968): 55–75.

————. *Image Formation and Cognition*. New York: Appleton, 1970.

————. "Controls of Visual Imagery and Therapeutic Intervention." In *The Power of Human Imagination*, edited by J. L. Singer and K. S. Pope. New York: Plenum, 1978.

Hultkrantz, A. "A Definition of Shamanism." *Temenos* 9 (1973): 25–37.

Humphrey, M. E., and Zangwill, O. L. "Cessation of Dreaming after Brain Injury." *Journal of Neurology, Neurosurgery, and Psychiatry* 14 (1951): 322–325.

Ingelfinger, F. J. "The Physicians Contribution to the Health System." *New England Journal of Medicine*, 295 (Sept. 2, 1976): 565–566.

Jackson, J. H. "On Right or Left-Sided Spasm at the Onset of Epileptic Paroxysms, and on Crude Sensation Warnings and Elaborate Mental States." *Brain* 3 (1980): 192–206.

Jacobsen, C. F. "Studies of Cerebral Function in Primates: 1. The functions of the frontal associations areas in monkeys." *Comparative Psychology Monographs*. 13 (1936): 3–60.

Jacobsen, E. "Electrical Measurements of Neuromuscular States During Mental Activities: Imagination of Movement Involving Skeletal Muscle." *American Journal of Physiology* 91 (1929): 597–608.

Jaffe, D. T., and Bresler, D. E. "Guided Imagery: Healing Through the Mind's Eye." In *Imagery: Its Many Dimensions and Applications*, edited by J. E. Shorr; G. E. Sobel; P. Robin; and J. A. Connella. New York: Plenum, 1980.

James, W. *The Varieties of Religious Experience*. New York: Collier Books, 1961.

Janet, P. *Nervoses et Idees Fixes*. Paris: Alcan, 1898.

Jellinek, A. "Spontaneous Imagery: A New Psychotherapeutic Approach." *American Journal of Psychotherapy* 3 (1949): 372–391.

Jilek, W. G. *Salish Indian Mental Health and Culture Change: Psycho Hygienic and Therapeutic Aspects of the Guardian Spirit Ceremonial*. Toronto and Montreal: Holt, Rinehart & Winston of Canada, 1974.

——. *Indian Healing*. Blaine, Wash.: Hancock House, 1982.

Jilek-Aall, L. *Call Mama Doctor*. Seattle, Wash.: Hancock House, 1979.

Johannes, A. "Many Medicines in One: Curing in the Eastern Highlands of Papua New Guinea." *Culture, Medicine, and Psychiatry* (Mar. 4, 1980): 43–70.

John, E. R., and Killam, K. F. "Electrophysiological Correlates of Avoidance Conditioning in the Cat." *Journal of Pharmacology and Experimental Therapeutics* 125 (1959): 252–274.

Johnson, J. E. "Effects of Accurate Expectations about Sensations on the Sensory and Distress Components of Pain." *Journal of Personality and Social Psychology* 27 (1973): 261–275.

——.; Rice, V. H.; Fuller, S. S.; and Endress, M. P. "Sensory Information Instruction in a Coping Strategy, and Recovery from Surgery." *Research in Nursing and Health*. 1(1) (1978): 4–17.

Jordan, C. S. "Mental Imagery and Psychotherapy: European Approaches." In *The Potential of Fantasy and Imagination*, edited by A. A. Sheikh and J. T. Shaffer. New York: Brandon House, 1979.

——, and Lenington, K. T. "Psychological Correlates of Eidetic

Imagery and Induced Anxiety." *Journal of Mental Imagery* 3(1979): 31–42.

Jung, C. G. "The Structure and Dynamics of the Psyche." In *Collected Works*, vol. 8. Translated by R. F. C. Hull. Princeton: Princeton University Press, 1960. (Originally published in 1926.)

Kamiya, J. Material presented to the International Conference on Science and Shamanism, Esalen Institute, Big Sur, California, February, 1984.

Kanfer, F. H. "The Many Faces of Self-Control: or Behavior Modification Changes its Focus." In *Behavioral Self Management: Strategies, Techniques and Outcomes*, edited by R. B. Stuart. New York: Brunner/Mazel, 1977.

Kazdin, A. E., and Wilcoxin, L. A. "Systematic Desensitization and Non-Specific Treatment Effects: A Methodological Evaluation." *Psychological Bulletin* 83 (1975): 5.

Kazner, M. "Image Formation During Free Association." *Psychoanalytic Quarterly* 27 (1958): 465–484.

Kendall, L. "Supernatural Traffic: East Asian Shamanism." *Culture, Medicine, and Psychiatry* 5 (1981): 171–191.

Kenner, C., and Achterberg, J. "Non-Pharmacologic Pain Relief for Patients." Presented to the American Burn Association Annual Meetings, New Orleans, La., April, 1983. (Winner, John A. Moncrief Award, Best Scientific Paper, Allied Health Category.)

Kiester, E. "The Playing Fields of the Mind." *Psychology Today* 18 (July, 1984): 18–24.

Kleinman, A. "Some Issues for a Comparative Study of Medical Healing." *International Journal of Social Psychiatry* 19(159) (1973): 159.

———, and Sung, L. H. "Why Do Indigenous Practitioners Successfully Heal?" *Social Sciences and Medicine* 13B (1979): 7–26.

Klopfer, B. "Psychological Variables in Human Cancer." *Journal of Projective Techniques* 21 (1957): 331–340.

Kosbab, F. P. "Imagery Techniques in Psychiatry." *Archives of General Psychiatry* 31 (1974): 283–290.

Kramer, H., and Sprenger, J. *The Malleus Maleficarum*. Translated by Rev. Montague Summers. London: Pushkin Press, 1928. Original writing: 1486.

Kraus, R. F. "A Psychoanalytic Interpretation of Shamanism." *The Psychoanalytic Review* 591 (1972): 19–32.

Kreig, M. B. *Green Medicine: The Search for Medicines that Heal*. New York: Bantam, 1966.

Kretschmer, W. "Meditative Techniques in Psychotherapy." In *Altered States of Consciousness*, edited by C. Tart. New York: Wiley, 1969.

Krieger, D. *Therapeutic Touch: How to Use Your Hands to Help or Heal*. Englewood Cliffs, N. J.: Prentice-Hall, 1979.

Krippner, S., and Villoldo, A. *The Realms of Healing*. Milbrae, Ca.: Celestial Arts, 1976.

LaBarre, W. *The Ghost Dance: Origins of Religion*. New York: Delta, 1972.

———. *The Peyote Cult*. New Haven: Yale University Press, 1938.

———. "Shamanic Origins of Religion and Medicine." *Journal of Psychedelic Drugs* II, 1–2 (1979): 7–11.

Laing, R. D. *The Politics of Experience*. New York: Ballantine, 1967.

Landy, D., ed. *Culture, Disease and Healing: Studies in Medical Anthropology.* New York: Macmillan, 1977.

Lashley, K. "In Search of the Engram." *Symposium for the Society of Experimental Biology* 4 (1950): 425–482.

LaViolette, F. E. *The Struggle for Survival: Indian Cultures and the Protestant Ethic in British Columbia.* Toronto: University of Toronto Press, 1961.

Lazarus, A. A., and Abramovitz, A. "The Use of 'Emotive Imagery' in the Treatment of Children's Phobias." *Journal of Mental Science* 108 (1962): 191–195.

Lea, H. C. *Materials Toward a History of Witchcraft, vol. 1–3.* Arranged and edited by Arthur C. Howland. New York: Thomas Yoseloff, 1957.

Leaf, A. "Every Day is a Gift When You Are Over 100." *National Geographic Magazine* 143 (1973): 93–118.

LeShan, L., *The Medium, the Mystic, and the Physicist.* New York: Ballantine Books, 1975.

———. *The Mechanic and the Gardener.* New York: Holt, Rinehart & Winston, 1982.

Lesser, I. M. "A Review of the Alexithymia Concept." *Psychosomatic Medicine* 32 (1981): 531–543.

Leuner, H. "Guided Affective Imagery: An Account of Its Development." *Journal of Mental Health* 1 (1977): 73–92.

———. "Basic Principles and Therapeutic Efficacy of Guided Affective Imagery." In *The Power of Human Imagination,* edited by J. L. Singer and K. S. Pope. New York: Plenum, 1978.

Levine, J. D.; Gordon, N. C.; and Fields, H. L. "The Mechanism of Placebo Analgesia." *The Lancet,* Sept. 23, 1978, pp. 654–657.

Levy, J.; Trevarthen, C.; and Sperry, R. W. "Perception of Bilateral Chimeric Figures Following Hemispheric Deconnection." *Brain* 95 (1972): 61–78.

Lichstein, K. L., and Lipshitz, E. "Psychophysiological Effects of Noxious Imagery: Prevalence and Prediction." *Behavior Research and Therapy* 20 (1982): 339–345.

Lilly, J. C. *The Center of the Cyclone: An Autobiography of Inner Space.* New York: Julian, 1972.

———. *The Deep Self.* New York: Simon and Schuster, 1977.

Lipkin, S. "The Imagery Collage and its Use in Psychotherapy." *Psychotherapy: Theory, Research, and Practice* 2 (1970): 238–242.

Lipowski, Z. J. "Psychosomatic Medicine in the Seventies: An Overview." *The American Journal of Psychiatry* 134: 3 (1977): 233–238.

Locke, S. E. "Stress Adaptation and Immunity: Studies in Humans." *General Hospital Psychiatry* 4 (1982): 49–58.

———, and Horning-Rohan, M. *Mind and Immunity: Behavioral Immunology, An Annotated Bibliography 1976–1982.* New York: Institute for the Advancement of Health, 1983.

Loeb, E. M. "The Shaman of Niue." *American Anthropologist* 26 (1924): 393–402.

Lommel, A. *Shamanism.* New York: McGraw Hill, 1967.

Lorr, M.; McNair, D. M.; and Weinstein, G. H. "Early Effects of Librium Used with Psychotherapy." *Journal of Psychiatric Research* 1 (1962): 257–270.

Lowie, R. H. *Primitive Religion*. London: Routledge & Sons, 1925.

Luria, A. *The Mind of a Mnemonist*. New York: Basic Books, 1968.

Luthe, W. *Autogenic Therapy*, vol. 1–7. New York: Grune & Stratton, 1969.

Lyman, B.; Bernardin, S.; and Thomas, S. "Frequency of Imagery in Emotional Experience." *Perceptual and Motor Skills* 50 (1980): 1159–1162.

Lyons, A. S., and Petrucelli, R. J. *Medicine: An Illustrated History*. New York: Harry N. Abrams, Inc., 1978.

Majno, G. *The Healing Hand: Man and Wound in the Ancient World*. Cambridge: Harvard University Press, 1975.

Maple, E. *Magic, Medicine, and Quackery*. New York: A. S. Barnes & Co., 1968.

McMahon, C. E. "The Role of Imagination in the Disease Process: Pre-Cartesian History." *Psychological Medicine* 6 (1976): 179–184.

Meichenbaum, D. *Cognitive-Behavioral Modification: An Integrative Approach*. New York: Plenum, 1977.

———. "Why Does Using Imagery in Psychotherapy Lead to Change?" In *The Power of Human Imagination*, edited by J. L. Singer and K. S. Pope. New York: Plenum, 1978.

Melzack, R., and Wall, P. D. "Pain Mechanism: A New Theory." *Science* 150 (1965): 971–979.

Meyer, A., and Beck, E. *Prefrontal Leucotomy and Related Operations: Anatomic Aspects of Success or Failure*. Springfield, Ill.: Charles C. Thomas, 1954.

Milner, B. "Brain Mechanisms Suggested by Studies of Temporal Lobes." In *Brain Mechanisms Underlying Speech and Language*, edited by F. L. Darley. New York: Grune & Stratton, 1968, pp. 122–145.

———. "Interhemispheric Differences in the Localization of Psychological Process in Man." *British Medical Bulletin* 27 (1971): 272–277.

Morrell, F., and Jasper, H. H. "Electrographic Studies of the Formation of Temporary Connections in the Brain." *Electroencephalography and Clinical Neurophysiology* 8 (1956): 201–215.

Morrison, J. K. "Emotive Reconstruction Therapy. A Short-Term Psychotherapeutic Use of Mental Imagery." In *Imagery: Its Many Dimensions and Applications*, edited by J. E. Shorr; G. E. Soble; P. E. Robin; and J. A. Connella. New York: Plenum, 1980.

Munn, H. "The Mushroom of Language." In *Hallucinogens and Shamanism*, edited by M. Harner. New York: Oxford University Press, 1973.

Murray, M. *The Witch Cult in Western Europe*. Oxford: Oxford University Press, 1921.

Nauta, W. J. H. "Some Efferent Connections of the Prefrontal Cortex in the Monkey." In *The Frontal Granular Cortex and Behavior*, edited by J. M. Warren and K. Akert. New York: McGraw-Hill, 1964.

Neher, A. "Auditory Driving Observed with Scalp Electrodes in Normal Subjects." *EEG and Clinical Neurophysiology* 13 (1961): 449–451.

———. "A Physiological Explanation of Unusual Behavior in Ceremonies Involving Drums." *Human Biology* 34 (1962): 151–160.

Ness, R. C., and Wintrob, R. M. "Folk Healing: A Description and Synthesis." *American Journal of Psychiatry* 138:11 (1981), 1477–1481.

Newman, H. "Health Attitudes: Locus of Control and Religious Orientation." Master's thesis, University of Texas Health Science Center, School of Allied Health Sciences, Dallas, 1983.

Noel, D. C. *Seeing Castaneda: Reactions to the "Don Juan" Writings of Carlos Castaneda*. New York: G. P. Putnam's Sons, 1976.

Nolen, W. *Healing: A Doctor in Search of a Miracle*. Random House, 1974.

Noll, R. "Shamanism and Schizophrenia: A State-Specific Approach to the 'Schizophrenia Metaphor' of Shamanic States." *American Ethnologist* 10(3)(1983): 443–459.

Nordland, O. "Shamanism as an Experience of the 'Unreal.'" In *Studies of Shamanism*, edited by C. M. Edsman. Stockholm: Almquist & Wiksell, 1967.

Olton, D. S., and Noonberg, A. R. *Biofeedback: Clinical Applications in Behavioral Medicine*. Englewood Cliffs: Prentice Hall, 1980.

Ornish, D. *Stress, Diet and Your Heart*. New York: Holt, Rinehart & Winston, 1982.

Osler, W. *The Evolution of Modern Medicine*. New Haven: Yale University Press, 1921.

Oyle, I. *Magic, Mysticism and Modern Medicine*. Millbrae, Ca.: Celestial Arts, 1976.

———. *Time, Space and the Mind*. Millbrae, Ca.: Celestial Arts, 1976.

———. *The New American Medical Show*. Santa Cruz: Unity Press, 1979.

Page, J. *Blood: The River of Life*. Washington, D.C.: U.S. News Books, 1981.

Peavey, B. S. "Biofeedback Assisted Relaxation: Effects on Phagocytic Immune Function." Ph.D. dissertation, North Texas State University, Denton, Texas, 1982.

Pelletier, K. *Mind as Healer, Mind as Slayer*. New York: Dell, 1977.

Penfield, W., and Perot, P. "The Brain's Record of Auditory and Visual Experience." *Brain* 86 (1963): 595–596.

Perls, F. *Gestalt Therapy Verbatim*. New York: Bantam, 1970.

Perry, J. W. "Reconstitutive Process in the Psychopathology of the Self." *Annals of the New York Academy of Sciences* 96 (1962): 853–876.

Peters, L. G., and Price-Williams, D. "Towards an Experiential Analysis of Shamanism." *American Ethnologist* 7 (1980): 398–418.

Philips, C., and Hunter, M. "The Treatment of Tension Headache—II. EMG 'Normality' and Relaxation." *Behavioral Research and Therapy* 19(1981): 499–507.

Pilkington, T. L. "The Coincidence of Rheumatoid Arthritis and Schizophrenia." *Journal of Nervous and Mental Disease* 124 (1956): 604–607.

Popov, A. A. "How Sereptic Djarvoskin of the Nganasans (Tavgi Samoyeds) Became a Shaman." Translated by Stephen P. Dunn. In *Popular Beliefs and Folklore Tradition in Siberia*, edited by Vilmos Diozeg. Bloomington, Ind.: Indiana University Press, 1968.

Pribram, K. *Languages of the Brain*. Monterey, Ca.: Brooks/Cole Pub. Co., 1971.

————. "Problems Concerning the Structure of Consciousness." In *Consciousness and the Brain*, edited by G. G. Globus et al. New York: Plenum, 1976.

————. "What the Fuss is All About." In *The Holographic Paradigm and Other Paradoxes*, edited by K. Wilber. Boulder: Shambhala, 1982.

Progroff, I. *The Symbolic and the Real.* New York: Julian Press, 1963.

————. "Waking Dream and Living Myth." In *Myths, Dreams and Religion*, edited by J. Campbell. New York: Dutton, 1970.

Rachman, S. *Phobias: Their Nature and Control.* Springfield, Ill.: Thomas, 1968.

Radin, P. *Primitive Religion.* New York: Viking, 1937.

Reed, G. F. "Sensory Deprivation." In *Aspects of Consciousness*, edited by G. Underwood and R. Stevens. London: Academic Press, in press.

Reichard, G. A. *Navaho Religion.* New York: Pantheon Books, Bollingen Foundation, 1950.

Reyher, J. "Spontaneous Visual Imagery: Implications for Psychoanalysis, Psychopathology and Psychotherapy." *Journal of Mental Imagery* 2 (1977): 253–274.

Risse, G. B. "Shamanism: The Dawn of a Healing Profession." *Wisconsin Medical Journal* 71 (1972): 18–23.

Rogers, M. P.; Dubey, D.; and Reich, P. "The Influence of the Psyche and the Brain on Immunity and Disease Susceptibility: A Critical Review." *Psychosomatic Medicine* 41 (1979): 147–165.

Rogers, S. "Shamans and Medicine Men." *CIBA Symposia* 4 (1942): 1202–1223.

Rothenberg, J., ed. *Technicians of the Sacred: A Range of Poetries From Africa, America, Asia, and Oceania.* Garden City, N.Y.: Doubleday, 1968.

Safer, M. A., and Leventhal, H. "Ear Differences in Evaluating Emotional Tones of Voice and Verbal Content." *Journal of Experimental Psychology: Human Perception and Performance* 3 (1977): 75–82.

Saland, L. C.; van Epps, D. E.; Ortiz, E.; and Samora, A. "Acute Injections of Opiate Peptides into the Rat Cerebral Ventricle: A Macrophage-like Cellular Response." *Brain Research Bulletin* 10 (1983): 523–528.

Salter, A. *Conditioned Reflex Therapy.* New York: Farrar & Straus, 1949.

Samuels, A. Material presented at a conference entitled "Beyond the Relaxation Response: Self-Regulation Mechanisms and Clinical Strategies," sponsored by UCLA Extension, Los Angeles, California. October 26–28, 1984.

Samuels, M., and Bennett, H. *The Well Body Book.* New York: Random House-Bookworks, 1973.

————, and ————. *Be Well.* New York: Random House-Bookworks, 1974.

————, and Samuels, N. *Seeing with the Mind's Eye.* New York: Random House-Bookworks, 1975.

Saphir, J. R.; Gold, A.; Giambrone, J. et al. "Voodoo Poisoning in Buffalo, New York." *Journal of the American Medical Association* 202: 437–438, 1967.

Saretsky, T. *Active Techniques and Group Psychotherapy*. New York: Jason Aronson, 1977.

Schleifer, S. J.; Keller, S. E.; McKegney, F. P.; and Stein, M. "Bereavement and Lymphocyte Function." Paper presented at annual meeting, *American Psychiatric Association*, San Francisco, 1980.

Schneider, J.; Smith, C. W.; and Whitcher, S. "The Relationship of Mental Imagery to White Blood Cell (Neutrophil) Function: Experimental Studies of Normal Subjects." Uncirculated Mimeograph. Michigan State University, College of Medicine, East Lansing, Mich., 1983.

Schultz, J. H., and Luthe, W. *Autogenic Training: A Physiological Approach to Psychotherapy*. New York: Grune & Stratton, 1969.

Schwartz, G. E.; Weinberger, D. A.; and Singer, J. A. "Cardiovascular Differentiation of Happiness, Sadness, Anger, and Fear: Imagery and Exercise." *Psychosomatic Medicine* 43 (1981): 343–364.

Segal, J. "Biofeedback as a Medical Treatment." *Journal of the American Medical Association* 232 (April, 14, 1975): 179–180.

Seligman, M. E. P. *Helplessness*. San Francisco: W. H. Freeman & Co., 1975.

Selye, H. *The Stress of Life*. New York: McGraw-Hill, 1956.

Service, E. R. *A Profile of Primitive Culture*. New York: Harper & Brothers, 1958.

Shaw, W. A. "The Relation of Muscular Action Potentials to Imaginal Weight Lifting." *Archives of Psychology* (1940): 247–250.

Sheehan, P. W. "Hypnosis and Processes of Imagination." In *Hypnosis: Developments in Research and New Perspectives*, edited by E. Fromm, and R. E. Shor. New York: Aldine, 1979.

Sheikh, A., ed. *Imagery: Current Theory, Research and Application*. New York: Wiley, 1983.

———, and Jordan, C. S. "Clinical Uses of Mental Imagery." In *Imagery: Current Theory, Research and Application*, edited by A. Sheikh. New York: Wiley, 1983.

———, and Shaffer, J. T., eds. *The Potential of Fantasy and Imagination*. New York: Brandon House, 1979.

Sherrington, C. S. *Man on His Nature*. London: Cambridge University Press, 1940.

Shorr, J. E. *Psycho-Imagination Therapy: The Integration of Phenomenology and Imagination*. New York: Intercontinental Medical Book Corp., 1972.

———, Sobel, G. E.; Robin, P.; and Connella, J. A., eds. *Imagery: Its Many Dimensions and Applications*. New York: Plenum, 1980.

Silverman, J. "Shamanism and Acute Schizophrenia." *American Anthropologist* 69 (1967): 21–31.

Simonton, O. C.; Simonton, S.; and Creighton, J. *Getting Well Again*. Los Angeles: Tarcher, 1978.

Singer, J. S. *Imagery and Daydream Methods in Psychotherapy and Behavior Modification*. New York: Academic Press, 1974.

———, and Pope, K. S., eds. *The Power of the Human Imagination*. New York: Plenum, 1978.

Siskind, J. "Visions and Cures among the Sharanahua." In *Hallu-

cinogens and Shamanism, edited by M. Harner. New York: Oxford University Press, 1973.

Smith, C. W.; Schneider, J.; Minning, C.; and Whitcher, S. "Imagery and Neutrophil Function Studies: A Preliminary Report." Prepublication and personal communication. Michigan State University, Dept. of Psychiatry, 1981.

Sommers, F. "Dualism in Descartes: The Logical Ground." In *Descartes,* edited by M. Hooker. Baltimore: Johns Hopkins University Press, 1978.

Spanos, N.; Horton, C.; and Chaves, J. "The Effects of Two Cognitive Strategies on Pain Threshold." *Journal of Abnormal Psychology* 84 (1975): 677–681.

Sperry, R. W., and Gazzaniga, M. S. "Language Following Surgical Disconnection of the Hemispheres." In *Brain Mechanisms Underlying Speech and Language,* edited by F. L. Darley. New York: Grune & Stratton, 1967, pp. 108–121.

Stampfl, T., and Lewis, D. "Essentials of Therapy: A Learning Theory-Based Psychodynamic Behavioral Therapy." *Journal of Abnormal Psychology* 72 (1967): 496–503.

Stat, D. K. "Ancient Sound: The Whistling Vessels of Peru." *El Quarterly Journal of the Museum of New Mexico* 85 (1979): 2--7.

Stein, M.; Schiavi, R.; and Camerino, M. "Influence of Brain and Behavior on the Immune System." *Science* 191 (1976): 435–440.

Steinberg, S. "Endorphins: New Types and Sweet Links." *Science News* 124 (1983): 136.

Stoddart, A. M. *Life of Paracelsus.* London, 1911.

Strosahl, K. D., and Ascough, J. S. "Clinical Uses of Mental Imagery: Experimental Foundations, Theoretical Misconceptions, Research Issues." *Psychological Bulletin* 89 (1981): 422–438.

Suedfeld, P. *Restricted Environmental Stimulation.* New York: Wiley-Interscience, 1980.

————, and Borrie, R. A. "Altering States of Consciousness through Sensory Deprivation." In *Expanding Dimensions of Consciousness,* edited by A. A. Sugerman and R. E. Tarter. New York: Springer, 1978.

Suskind, J. "Visions and Cures Among the Sharanahua." In *Hallucinogens and Shamanism,* edited by M. Harner. New York: Oxford University Press, 1973.

Tart, C. T. "A Psychophysiological Study of Out-of-the-Body Experiences in Selected Subjects." *Journal of the American Society for Physical Research,* vol. 62 (January 1968): 1–16.

————. *States of Consciousness.* New York: E. P. Dutton, 1975.

Tenzel, J. H. "Shamanism and Concepts of Disease in a Mayan Indian Community." *Psychiatry* 33 (1970): 372–380.

Thomas, L. "On Warts." Chapter in *The Medusa and the Snail.* Toronto, New York, and London: Bantam Books, 1980.

Torrey, E. F. "What Western Psychotherapists Can Learn from Witchdoctors." *American Journal of Orthopsychiatry* 42: 1 (1972): 69–76.

Trestman, R. L. "Imagery, Coping and Physiological Variables in Adult Cancer Patients." Ph.D. dissertation, University of Tennessee, Knoxville, Tenn., 1981.

Trevor-Roper, H. R. *The European Witch-Craze of the Sixteenth and Seventeenth Centuries and Other Essays.* New York: Harper Torch Books, 1969.

Tucker, D. M.; Roth, R. S.; Arneson, B. A.; and Buckingham, T. M. "Right Hemisphere Activation during Stress." *Neuropyschologia,* 15 (1977): 697–700.

Underhill, E. *Mysticism,* 4th ed. London: Methuen and Co., 1912.

van Heerden, P. J. *The Foundation of Empirical Knowledge.* N. V. Uitgeverij Wistik-Wassenaar, the Netherlands, 1968.

Volgyesi, F. A. "School for Patients. Hypnosis-Therapy and Psychoprophylaxis." *British Journal of Medical Hypnosis* 5 (1954): 8–17.

Wasson, R. G. *Divine Mushroom of Immortality.* Ethno-Mycological Studies, No. 1. New York: Harcourt, Brace, Jovanovich, 1968.

Waterman, T. T. "The Paraphernalia of the Cuwamish 'Spirit-Canoe' Ceremony." *Indian Notes,* Museum of the American Indian, 1930.

Weatherhead, L. D. *Psychology, Religion and Healing.* New York: Abingdon-Cokesbury Press, 1951.

Weisburd, S. "Food for Mind and Mood." *Science News* 125 (1984): 216–219.

Wheeler, J.; Thorne, K. S.; and Misner, C. *Gravitation.* San Francisco: Freeman, 1973.

White, K. D. "Salivation: The Significance of Imagery in its Voluntary Control." *Psychophysiology* 15, 3 (1978): 196–203.

Wike, J. A. "Modern Spirit Dancing of Northern Puget Sound." Unpublished Master's thesis, University of Washington, Dept. of Anthropology, Seattle, Wash., 1941.

Wilber, K. *The Atman Project.* Wheaton, Ill.: Quest, 1980.

———, ed. *The Holographic Paradigm and Other Paradoxes.* Boulder: Shambhala, 1982.

Wildschut, W. "Crow Indian Medicine Bundles." In *Museum of the American Indian,* edited by J. C. Ewers. New York: Heye Foundation, 1975.

Williams, T. A. *Dreads and Besetting Fears.* Boston: Little, Brown, 1923.

Wissler, C. *The American Indian.* New York: Oxford University Press, 1931.

Wolf, S. "Effects of Suggestion and Conditioning on the Action of Chemical Agents in Human Subjects: The Pharmacology of Placebos." *Journal of Clinical Investigation* 29 (1950): 100–109.

Wolpe, J. *Psychotherapy by Reciprocal Inhibition.* Stanford: Stanford University Press, 1958.

———. *The Practice of Behavior Therapy.* New York: Pergamon, 1969.

Wolpin, M. "Guided Imagining to Reduce Avoidance Behavior." *Psychotherapy: Theory, Research and Practice* 6 (1969): 122–124.

Worthington, E. L., Jr. "The Effects of Imagery Content, Choice of Imagery Content, and Self-Verbalization on the Self-Control of Pain." *Cognitive Therapy and Research* 2 (1978): 225–240.

Wybran, J.; Appelbrrom, T.; Famaey, J. D. et al. "Suggestive Evidence for Receptors for Morphine and Methionine-Enkephalin on Normal Human Blood T-Lymphocytes." *Journal of Immunology* 123 (1979): 1068–1070.

Yanouski, A., and Fogel, M. L. "Some Diagnostic and Therapeutic Implications of Visual Imagery Reactivity." *Journal of Mental Imagery* 2 (1978): 301–302.

Zilboorg, G. *The Medicine Man and the Witch during the Renaissance.* New York: Cooper Square, 1969.

Zubek, J.; Welch, C.; and Saunders, M. "Electroencephalographic Changes During and After 14 Days of Perceptual Deprivation." *Science* 139 (1963): 490–492.

Zukerman, M. "Hallucinogens, Reported Sensations, and Images." In *Sensory Deprivation: Fifteen Years of Research,* edited by J. P. Zubek. New York: Appleton-Century Crofts, 1969.

Index

Also in New Science Library

Awakening the Heart: *East/West Approaches to Psychotherapy and the Healing Relationship,* by John Welwood.

Beyond Illness: *Discovering the Experience of Health,* by Larry Dossey, M.D.

Fisherman's Guide: *A Systems Approach to Creativity and Organization,* Robert Campbell.

The Holographic Paradigm and Other Paradoxes, edited by Ken Wilber.

Jungian Analysis, edited by Murray Stein. Introduction by June Singer.

No Boundary: *Eastern and Western Approaches to Personal Growth,* by Ken Wilber.

Order Out of Chaos: *Man's New Dialogue with Nature,* by Ilya Prigogine and Isabelle Stengers. Foreword by Alvin Toffler.

Perceiving Ordinary Magic: *Science and Intuitive Wisdom,* by Jeremy W. Hayward.

Quantum Questions: *Mystical Writings of the World's Great Physicists,* edited by Ken Wilber.

A Sociable God: *Toward a New Understanding of Religion,* by Ken Wilber.

Space, Time and Medicine, by Larry Dossey, M.D.

The Sphinx and the Rainbow: *Brain, Mind and Future Vision,* by David Loye.

Staying Alive: *The Psychology of Human Survival,* by Roger Walsh, M.D.

The Tao of Physics: *An Exploration of the Parallels between Modern Physics and Eastern Mysticism,* second edition, revised and updated, by Fritjof Capra.

Up from Eden: *A Transpersonal View of Human Evolution,* by Ken Wilber.

The Wonder of Being Human: *Our Brain and Our Mind,* by Sir John Eccles and Daniel N. Robinson.